GET
IT
DONE

BRADLEY
SIMMONDS

GET
IT
DONE

MY PLAN, YOUR GOAL:
60 Recipes & Workouts for
a Fit, Lean Body

HQ

HQ
An imprint of HarperCollins*Publishers* Ltd
1 London Bridge Street
London SE1 9GF

10 9 8 7 6 5 4 3 2 1

First published in Great Britain by HQ
An imprint of HarperCollins*Publishers* Ltd 2018

ISBN 978-0-00-822272-7

Photography: Glen Burrows
Food styling: Lizzie Kamenetzky
Prop styling: Morag Farquhar
Design: Manisha Patel
Senior Commissioning Editor: Rachel Kenny
Project Editor: Sarah Hammond
Head of Design: Louise McGrory

Our policy is to use papers that are natural, renewable
and recyclable products and made from wood grown
in sustainable forests. The logging and manufacturing
processes conform to the legal environmental regulations
of the country of origin. For more information visit:
www.harpercollins.co.uk/green

Printed and bound in Italy by Rotolito S.p.A.

CONTENTS

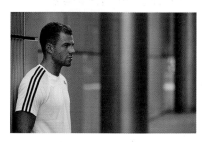

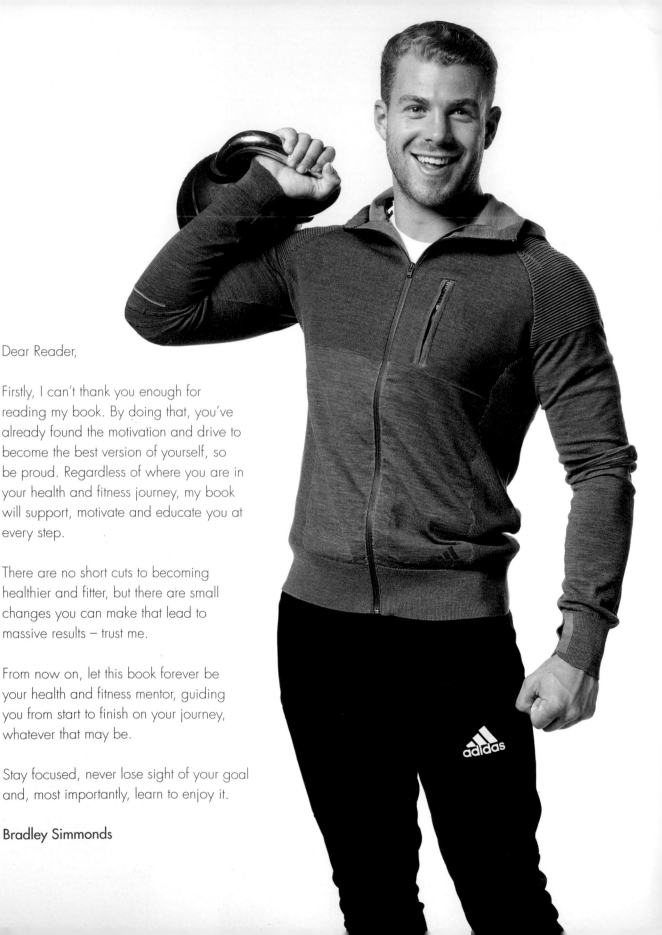

Dear Reader,

Firstly, I can't thank you enough for reading my book. By doing that, you've already found the motivation and drive to become the best version of yourself, so be proud. Regardless of where you are in your health and fitness journey, my book will support, motivate and educate you at every step.

There are no short cuts to becoming healthier and fitter, but there are small changes you can make that lead to massive results – trust me.

From now on, let this book forever be your health and fitness mentor, guiding you from start to finish on your journey, whatever that may be.

Stay focused, never lose sight of your goal and, most importantly, learn to enjoy it.

Bradley Simmonds

INTRODUCTION

I don't want *Get It Done* to just be a healthy recipe book. I want it to be a resource that helps you to figure out exactly what you want to achieve, then takes you on a journey to making that goal a reality. Whether you want to lose weight, build muscle tone or simply lead a healthier and more balanced life, this book will provide you with the right tools.

SO WHY THIS BOOK?

I know there are lots of health and fitness books out there, so why pick up *Get It Done*? I'll tell you why:

Nutrition and fitness is my job. As a former professional sportsperson, now personal trainer, I've had access to the best nutritional and fitness advice out there since I was a kid. I know this area inside out, and I'm passionate about health and wellness.

I've been where you are. I've come back from career-halting injuries, weight gain, frustration and unhappiness all through eating the right food and moving the right way for my body and my goals.

Over 200,000 people follow me on Instagram @bradleysimmonds for fitness inspiration and motivation – so I reckon I must be doing something right!

I am uncompromising in my pursuit of health, fitness and wellbeing, and I will push you to be the same.

ABOUT ME

MY REALISATION

I didn't always want to be a personal trainer, in fact at school and growing up it didn't even cross my mind. As far as I was concerned I was a footballer and nothing else; I managed to get pretty far, playing for Chelsea FC and Queen's Park Rangers.

My last six months as a footballer were spent on the tranquil island country of Iceland, playing for ÍBV Vestmannaeyja. Iceland is one of the world's most beautiful places and the Icelanders' active lifestyles and love of fresh food really rubbed off on me. Now looking back, my time in Iceland marked a turning point in my career. It was also the first time I had lived away from home without a big group of friends and my huge family near by.

In my spare time, I explored the landscape and immersed myself in the culture of Iceland, which, incidentally, was recently voted the healthiest nation in the world. This didn't surprise me; with lobster and fish being their equivalent to our steak and chicken, Icelandic people have an extremely lean diet full of essential fats and omega 3.

I've always loved to cook, but my passion for cooking healthy food with good-quality produce began in Iceland. I lived with David James, ex Liverpool and England goalkeeper. He was pretty strict when it came to his diet, refusing my butter and Marmite on toast on cheat days. However, when it came to my super-lean chilli con carne, he couldn't refuse!

The healthy eating and active lifestyle got me my first ever six-pack. You may laugh, but this was a personal goal of mine! Now, with the knowledge I have, I've been able to maintain it. Don't get me wrong; it's definitely not easy, but when you want something enough, you find the motivation.

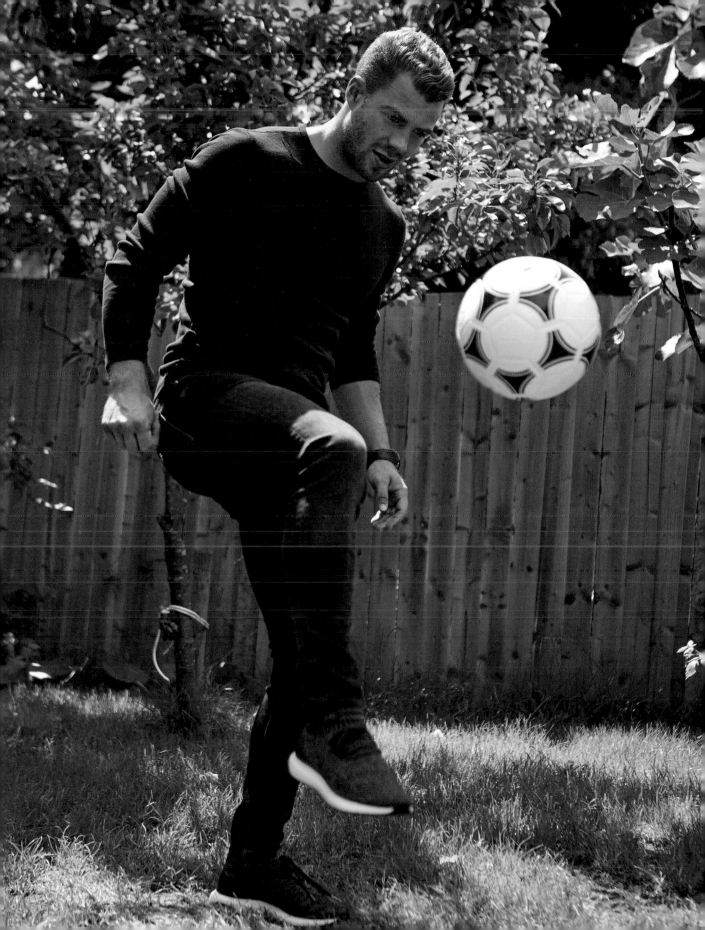

FOOTBALL 1 BRADLEY 0

My time as a footballer was amazing. From ages 7 to 19 I travelled across Italy, Spain, Portugal and Greece to France, Holland and Belgium and, naturally, I picked up the tactics of opposing teams – including how they fuelled themselves before a game! (My interest in health and fitness developed from there, but I'll come back to that later.)

This chapter came to an abrupt end when I suffered a couple of serious injuries: first an ACL tear in my knee, followed by a fractured ankle. These were huge setbacks, at a vital time in my career. At 20 years old I should have been playing first-team football, but instead I was looking at the four walls of a physio room. I was angry and frustrated with myself and my body. I'd always been fearless on the pitch – that was my strength – but that strength had ultimately been my undoing. I knew it was only a matter of time before I was replaced.

On top of that, I was losing motivation and my passion for football, particularly because I'd gone from exercising every day, to not exercising at all and not changing my eating habits. And – you guessed it – my body fat percentage increased. Nothing major, but I noticed it and I felt uncomfortable and frustrated. But instead of feeling sorry for myself, I did something about it.

I began working out in the gym, mainly upper body due to my injuries, and realised I couldn't eat what I wanted anymore. All the lessons on nutrition as a footballer really started to become useful, and I found myself educating my whole family – that's my mum, dad, two brothers James and Elliott and

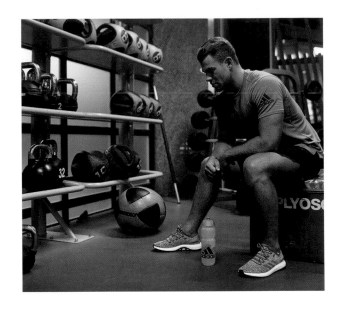

my sister Connie – on the best foods to eat and encouraged them to get more active, even if it was just power walking.

'THE BIGGEST DIFFERENCE FOR ME WAS MY WEIGHT. I LOST WEIGHT, ESPECIALLY AROUND MY MIDDLE AREA, AND HAVE BEEN ABLE TO KEEP IT OFF. I THINK THE HEALTHY SWAPS AND REDUCING THE AMOUNT OF SUGAR I ATE IS THE MAIN REASON.'
MY MUM

At that time, all six of us were living at home. Mum cooked dinner and it had to be quick, easy and not too expensive. So you can imagine it was a bit of a challenge to get us off our favourite white pasta, potatoes and white rice! My dad was the most resistant. He's pretty stubborn (like father, like son…) and didn't realise how bad his diet was until he wrote a food diary for me.

But I managed to persuade the gang to put in place small changes – like swapping white rice for brown rice and reducing portion sizes – that made a big difference. We also stopped buying white bread and stuck to sourdough or rye bread. At first the change was difficult. They were used to everything being so sweet, so the food seemed bland in comparison, but gradually my mum and dad realised these darker breads had more flavour than our previous family favourite white loaf and that we were less bloated and had a lot more energy. Further down the line, we made the switch to better vegetable and nut oils and substituted white potatoes for sweet potatoes or

root vegetables. More good fats and less starch in our diets made weight loss easier, and we began experimenting with herbs and spices. One of the factors that made the biggest obvious difference was reducing the amount of sugar in our diets. We cooked as much as we could from scratch to avoid added or hidden sugar. Sugar has more of an impact on your life than you realise, believe me.

'I ACTUALLY FEEL QUITE BAD FOR HOW MOODY I WAS. THE AMOUNT OF HEADACHES I WOULD GET WAS UNREAL, PROBABLY EVERY DAY. REMOVING REFINED SUGAR FROM MY DIET AND AVOIDING WHITE PASTA AND BREAD HAS ACTUALLY BEEN ESSENTIAL FOR MY WELLBEING, WEIGHT AND PERSONALITY.'
CONNIE, MY SISTER

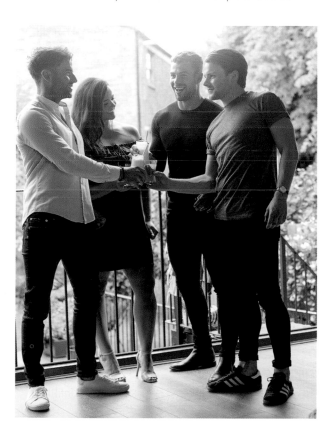

After a short while, I began to notice that my dad was in a much better mood and his skin had improved. My sister's mood swings had disappeared and as a whole the family was losing weight. Seeing how much my entire family benefitted from improving their diet and changing their ingrained unhealthy habits, I found a new passion: helping people transform their lives into healthier ones, starting with my own. That's when I googled 'How to be the best personal trainer'.

BECOMING A PERSONAL TRAINER

After years of being an athlete, I began my journey as a personal trainer in 2015, aged 20. While still recovering from my injuries and without a salary, I put all my life savings into a personal training course. I'm a strong believer that everything happens for a reason, so despite the horrific injuries, I'm now thankful for them as they've taken me on a journey that I love.

For me the marker of a good personal trainer is their ability to motivate their client and make them feel better in themselves and about their body. In a session with a client I'm serious and focused because that's what I expect my client to be. Nevertheless, my workouts are fun, varied and undoubtedly get results.

I really enjoy the social aspect of my job; nothing is instant and building relationships with my clients and the people I train with is a massive highlight of what I do. I've enjoyed many perks and have travelled to the most beautiful places, including Monaco, Dubai, Barbados and Arizona, training with interesting, inspiring people.

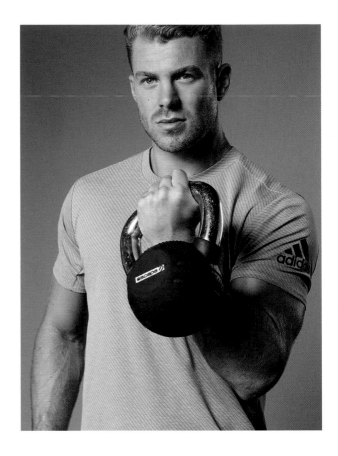

I WAS VERY RELUCTANT TO JOIN IN WITH THE SWAPS AND LIKED TO THINK I WASN'T ACTUALLY EATING THAT MUCH SUGAR. IT DEFINITELY IS AN ADDICTION. I STILL CRAVE SOMETHING SWEET AFTER DINNER BUT WE ALWAYS HAVE DARK CHOCOLATE IN THE FRIDGE FOR THAT.'

MY DAD

I love sharing my knowledge with clients and learning from others in the field. I've always believed that everyone you meet knows something you don't. This philosophy is a great one for the stubborn people out there; don't think you know best, we are always evolving.

It's definitely a lot more admirable when someone admits they can be healthier or can work harder. For me there is nothing worse than someone who is 'proud' to be unhealthy.

SOCIAL MEDIA CHANGED EVERYTHING

My first job was at Virgin Active Gym, Chiswick. I'd ride my dad's bike to and from work every day, then train clients all day. However, even though I was working as much as I possibly could, I knew I couldn't help everyone in the gym. But honestly, I really wanted to.

By watching people in the gym struggle with technique, fear creativity and clearly lack confidence, it gave me the idea to post fitness videos on my Instagram. That way I could help a lot more people and showcase my style of training. Some people laughed as it was such a new concept; others found it extremely useful and motivating.

My followers began to grow and I plucked up the courage to approach some more high-profile clients to gain credibility, exposure and to build my brand.

TRAINING CELEBRITY CLIENTS AND ATHLETES...

Made in Chelsea was the hit show at the time, so I contacted the female cast members offering free personal training sessions in exchange for exposure. Luckily, Sophie Hermann and the Watson sisters took up the offer and became my new clients. As my profile grew, my videos became more and more popular and people who were inspired by me and my style would tag me in their videos.

As my credibility and following increased from 20,000 to 60,000, I decided I wanted to focus on going back to my roots. It was important for me to train athletes because not only did I completely understand the damaging emotional, physical and financial repercussions of injuries on professional sportspeople, I now had a really comprehensive grasp of how to enhance their performance while preventing injury. This is when I began training John Terry and Theo Walcott.

TWO YEARS LATER...

Now, at 23, I've trained some of my personal sporting heroes and represented Adidas, Lucozade Sport, TAG Heuer, *Women's Health* magazine, *Men's Health* magazine and Maximuscle.

But even though I've had access to some of the most well-equipped gyms and state-of-the-art equipment, I've tried to stay true to my ethos that exercise can be done anywhere if you have the right mindset, and that's reflected on my Instagram.

I've experienced a whirlwind of emotions in the last couple of years, from the fear of failure to the excitement of a new challenge. My journey has proved to me that with the right attitude, outlook, and determination you can turn things round. I'm proof that even if you feel you have hit rock bottom, you can get up and you can go on to achieve amazing things.

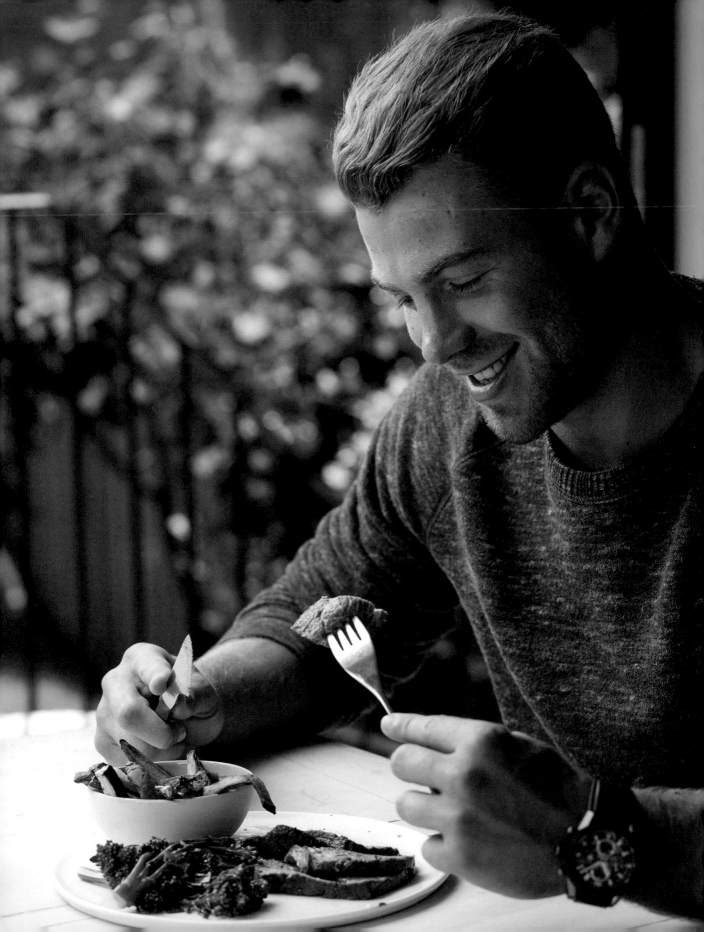

NOW TO YOU

MINDSET

Before you embark on your journey we are going to focus on your mindset. You can dream of having the best body in the world every night and think about it every day, but if you aren't focused, committed and determined to work for it, it will never happen. Not everything comes easy in life, but with a positive mental attitude you'll be surprised at how easy it can actually be.

Exercise doesn't have to take 60 minutes to be effective and you don't have to give up your social life to reach your goal. The sooner you make exercise and healthy eating a normal part of your daily routine, the better you'll feel and the easier it will be.

I hate when clients repeatedly cancel sessions or constantly moan. When it comes to your health, consistency should be viewed in a positive light, as it's essential to maintaining your goal. Don't get me wrong, initially it will require perseverance, but once you start noticing the changes you won't want to be anything but consistent.

BALANCE

Another key ingredient of realising your goal is balance. It's a word used commonly in the health and fitness industry, but often misunderstood.

For example, I used to think that because I was training every day as a footballer I could eat what I wanted. What I know now is that balance is about a VARIETY of nutrient-dense food so we get the vital vitamins and minerals needed for healthy body function, and CONSISTENCY of healthy habits. Regardless of what your goal is, the food we eat needs to provide us with more than just energy.

I love my food so much but I have to remember to occasionally rein it in because it doesn't matter how much exercise you do – if you're eating the wrong food, a poor diet will always catch up with you. So if you love treating yourself as much as you love sweating it out, you may have to rethink.

On the other hand, if you do no exercise at all and eat what you want (yes, even if you're one of the lucky ones who, from the outside, seems to get away with eating as you please), you need to wake up and start caring for your mind and body. A bad diet will be putting stress on your internal organs, it'll increase your cholesterol levels, and you'll be experiencing manufactured energy highs followed by sudden dips, not to mention how it'll be affecting your mood. In this book I will offer you clear guidance on how to find the right balance, depending on what it is you want to achieve.

PRIORITISING

We all have jobs, a social life, a home, hobbies and both family and friends to juggle. There's no doubt that you're busy, but no matter how busy you are, it's imperative that you make time to nourish and respect your body – even if this is at the expense of other things you feel you 'should' be doing. Your body carries you through your hectic schedule after all! For a lot of people, exercise and eating well isn't a priority but a chore. Put it this way: by prioritising your health, you're allowing yourself to enjoy your life for a lot longer and the juggling will become a lot easier.

In all honesty, there is no excuse. Exercise can be done anywhere and at any time and eating well only requires a little organisation and basic knowledge. Everyone can squeeze in a 30-minute workout at home when you get in from work or before you go to bed. It's certainly better than 30 minutes of TV, simply because of how good you feel afterwards. I'll demonstrate how you can do this later in the book! Even clients of mine who are mothers of young babies find new ways to exercise, such as squatting with a baby carrier strapped on their fronts or going for power walks around the park pushing the buggy. It is always possible.

DON'T GET DISTRACTED

With the health and fitness industry growing faster than ever before, we as a nation are becoming better educated about the importance of a balanced diet and exercise. Nevertheless, with so many faddy diets, super food myths and new food discoveries it is so easy to get caught up, confused and then unmotivated. Just like when everyone believed a fat-free diet was the way forward (it's not by the way)!

I like to keep things simple, realistic and to the point. I never over-complicate recipes and I certainly don't follow the crowd. I focus on what foods are right for me and my clients and what will help us get to where we want to be.

The same goes for exercise. There are so many forms of exercise to choose from and some will help you reach your goal more quickly than others. However, it is also just as important to find the exercise style that keeps you motivated. I'll be discussing exercise styles and finding your favourite exercise in the next chapters.

By figuring out early what foods and forms of exercise are right for you and your goal, formulating a plan and then sticking with that plan, you will feel mentally stronger and far less easily influenced.

BE HONEST WITH YOURSELF

Some of us are really good at knowing exactly where we need to improve and others get lulled into a false sense of security, telling themselves that they're happy with how they look and feel because they aren't quite ready to change. In my experience, most people who have got themselves out of that mindset and have accomplished their goals through training and healthy eating look back and realise they were not happy at all.

So being honest with yourself is a key factor in starting this journey. Let me ask you:

- Do you feel overweight?

- Are you lazy when it comes to your health?

- Do you hate having cellulite?

- Do you dislike your man boobs?

- Could you do more on a weekly basis to get fitter and stronger?

- Do you make excuses at every opportunity?

- Does the healthy eating always start tomorrow?

I know all about this through my sister and her journey, which I will be touching on shortly. Living with her gave me a real insight into the struggles she faced and the barriers she would put up whenever we discussed a healthier lifestyle.

Nevertheless, if you're reading my book I assume you've made the decision to change, which is such a big step.

NO EXCUSES

I have worked with clients from all walks of life, all with their own excuses.

If you are the 9–5 worker who grabs a coffee and a croissant on the way to work, followed by a meal deal or last night's leftover lasagne, with a few sneaky snacks in between, you're bound to feel tired. Or maybe you're the taxi driver parent (like mine used to be) who grabs a slice of toast smothered in butter and marmalade whilst your kids enjoy a bowl of cereal. Not forgetting the social bunnies who can't say no to a cocktail regardless of what day it is.

- 'After work I'm just too tired and sluggish to cook.'

- 'I deserve a treat at the end of the day.'

- 'Cooking healthy food that all the family will enjoy is really difficult.'

- 'I don't want to give up going out and having fun with my friends.'

Whoever you are, it is time to leave the excuses behind. Excuses are just a form of laziness. All they mean is you simply haven't discovered what works for you.

This book is packed full of realistic advice, taking into consideration people like you. So, be prepared for my no-nonsense approach to health and fitness, because the only way to achieve it is to **GET IT DONE.**

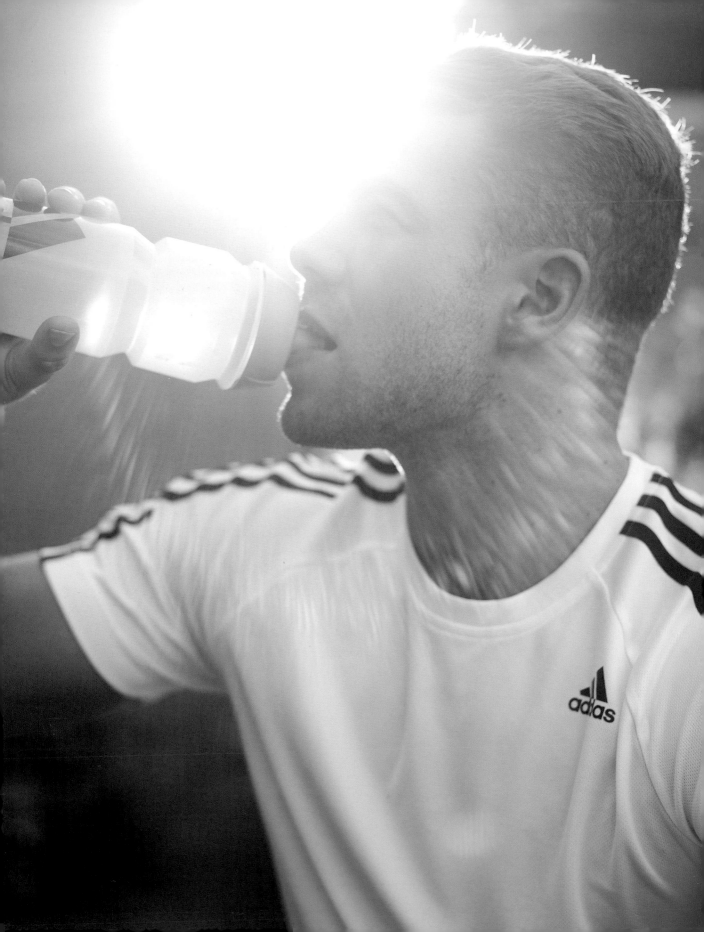

HOW THE BOOK WORKS...

This book has been structured to support you, from the start of your health and fitness journey right through to reaching your goal and maintaining all your hard work.

- You'll be defining your specific goal (or goals!), what you plan to achieve and how to achieve it in chapter 1, Realising Your Goal, whether that's weight-loss, toning, gaining lean muscle, improving your mental health and energy levels, or focusing on core strength.

- You'll discover new ways of exercising and how to enjoy it in chapter 2, Now Get moving, at home or in the gym.

- You'll cook delicious meals that are right for you in chapter 3, Fuel Your Fitness – from breakfast right through to dessert.

- You'll learn how to measure and maintain your hard work in chapter 4, Maintaining Your Goal.

- You'll be the best version of yourself.

It's time to look good and feel good and this book is all about doing it the right way.

LET'S GO

All I need from you is your determination and dedication – remember, it is all about your mindset. Lastly, don't let my no-nonsense approach put you off – you'll love me for it in the end! A bit of tough love never hurt nobody, so suck it up so you don't have to suck it in.

YOU DON'T HAVE TO BE GREAT TO START, BUT YOU HAVE TO START TO BE GREAT.

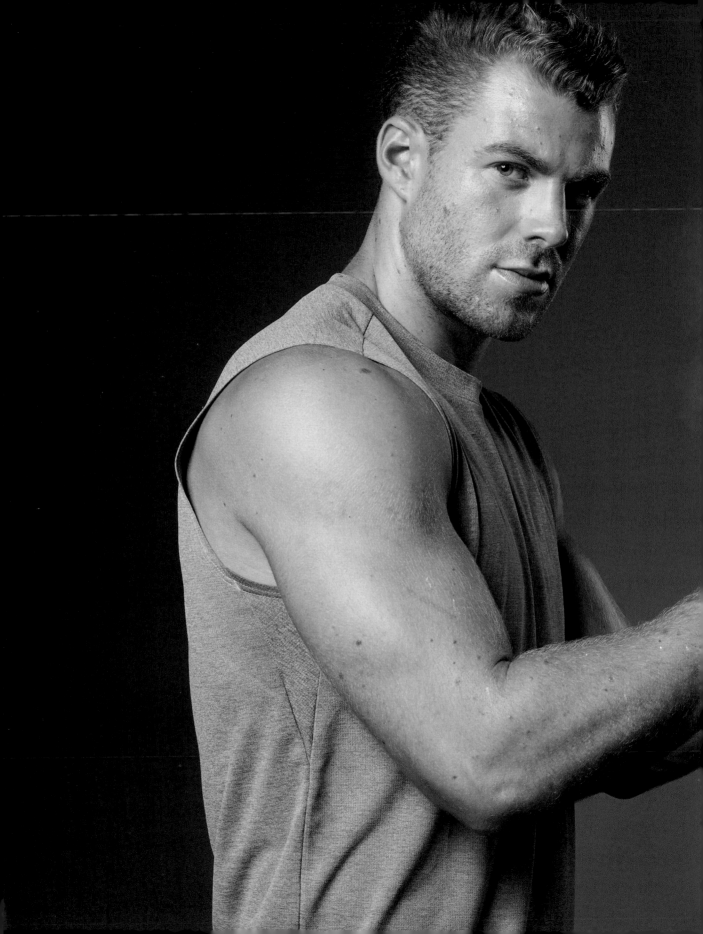

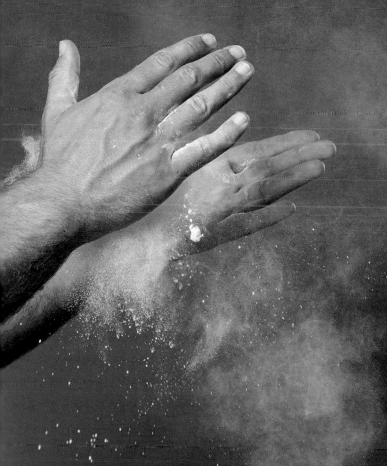

CHAPTER 1

REALISING YOUR GOAL

IT'S REALLY IMPORTANT TO FIGURE OUT WHY YOU'RE ON THIS JOURNEY, WHAT YOU WANT TO ACHIEVE AND WHY YOU WANT TO ACHIEVE IT, AS THAT WILL HELP MOTIVATE YOU WHEN YOU REALLY DON'T WANT TO GET OUT OF BED, WHEN IT'S RAINING AND COLD, OR WHEN ALL YOU WANT IS TO SLOB OUT ON THE SOFA FOR THE WEEKEND WITH A TUB OF ICE CREAM.

WHATEVER YOUR REASON FOR CHOOSING TO LIVE A HEALTHIER LIFESTYLE, YOUR AIMS IN EXERCISING AND EATING WELL WILL LIKELY FALL INTO ONE OF THE FIVE GOALS OUTLINED ON PAGES 24–49.

READ THROUGH THESE CAREFULLY – THE BENEFITS YOU'LL NOTICE, AND THE SOLUTION TO ACHIEVING THOSE GOALS – AND DECIDE WHICH ONE WILL MOTIVATE YOU THE MOST. TRY TO BE AS SPECIFIC AS POSSIBLE WHEN THINKING ABOUT THE TIME YOU WANT TO REACH YOUR GOAL IN, AND MAKE SURE IT'S EASILY MEASURABLE.

FOR EXAMPLE:

- **WEIGHT LOSS.** TO FIT INTO YOUR SIZE 10 JEANS AGAIN IN TIME FOR YOUR BIRTHDAY.

- **FEELING HAPPIER AND MORE ENERGETIC** BY THIS TIME NEXT MONTH, SO THAT YOU DON'T SLEEP THROUGH YOUR ALARM EVERY MORNING AND INSTEAD GET TO WORK EARLY AND LEAVE ON TIME, RATHER THAN FEELING GUILTY ABOUT COMING IN LATE AND STAYING LATER THAN YOU NEED.

- **STRENGTHENING YOUR CORE.** TO GET RID OF THE BACK PAIN BROUGHT ON FROM SITTING AT A DESK ALL DAY.

JOT YOUR GOAL DOWN SOMEWHERE YOU CAN SEE IT DAILY. ONCE YOU'VE RECORDED YOUR GOAL, THIS BOOK WILL GUIDE YOU TOWARDS MAKING THE RIGHT DECISIONS BY TAILORING MEALS, EXERCISES AND LIFESTYLE CHOICES AROUND THAT GOAL.

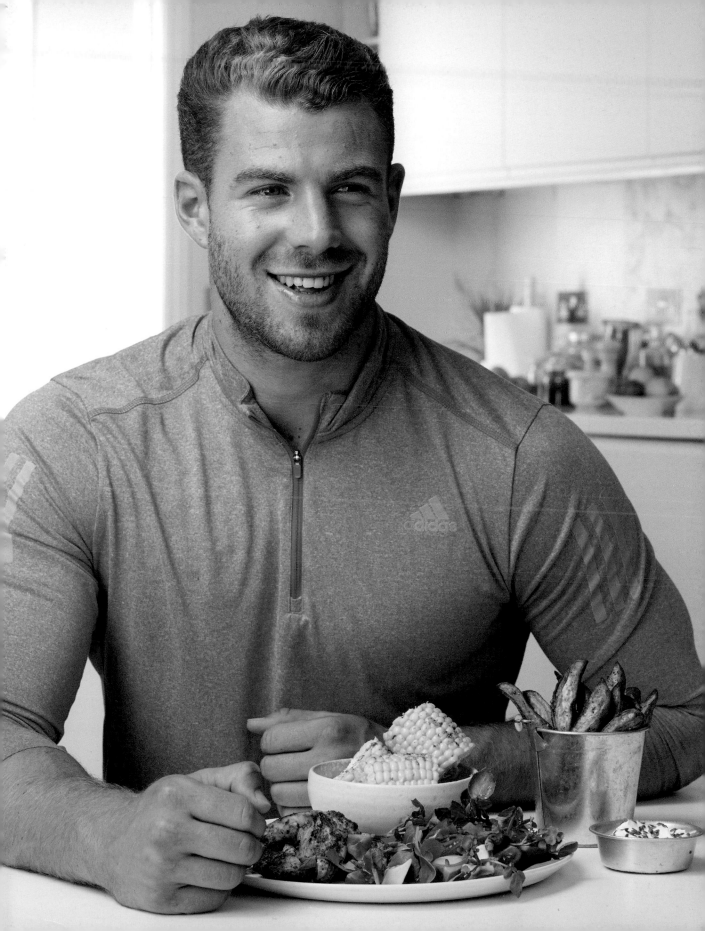

1 WEIGHT LOSS

Weight loss is a goal for hundreds of thousands of people everywhere. Many people struggle to ever reach their goal because bad habits and temptation always get the better of them. Some people starve themselves or over-exercise to lose weight quickly, but as this punishing lifestyle is unsustainable they can't keep the weight off, so their weight fluctuates, creating an unhealthy cycle. If this is you, then keep reading. My sister's journey may give you the inspiration you're lacking. Connie went from a size 16 to a healthy size 12 in just 12 weeks by following my food and fitness plan.

Connie loved sport throughout school and had never been overweight. But aged 18 she went to university, where she threw herself into the lifestyle of drinking and eating cheap processed food. She then got herself a 9–5 job when she graduated, where she sat at a desk (with a snack drawer) all day and, finally, she had a long-term boyfriend who wasn't healthy at the time either. She admits these were all contributing factors to her gradual weight gain over the last 5 years. Nevertheless, when it came to doing something about it she always had an excuse, the biggest one always being: 'I am perfectly happy the way I am'.

I knew she wasn't deep down. I knew she longed for her old body back. She would hide herself in big baggy tops, day or night, and never wanted full body pictures taken. She would have weeks or months of trying to lose weight, but nothing really lasted because she wasn't consistent. I had to figure out what would motivate my sister to lose weight so that she could become happier and healthier.

Connie had a year of stomach infections and in the end they became the trigger to her change of mindset. She was sick of feeling unhealthy and wanted to feel good again because it was affecting her mood and productivity at work. Once we established this, Connie was more willing to admit that she wanted to look and feel better.

THE SOLUTION
FOOD

1 CUT OUT SUGAR

One huge factor contributing to weight gain and obesity is sugar. Sugar has so many negative effects, mentally and physically. It is addictive and makes us fat! Studies have shown that sugar is even more addictive than illegal drugs like cocaine, yet sadly the majority of convenience foods, jars and snacks found in supermarkets and cupboards are riddled with it.

Sugar avoiding tips:

- Cook everything from scratch to avoid added sugar or hidden sugar.

- Empty all cupboards of sweet treats and processed foods.

- Don't go food shopping hungry – if you don't buy it, you can't eat it!

- Use sugar alternatives such as dried fruits or honey (in moderation).

- See sugar as something damaging to your body rather than a treat.

Many products that are FAT FREE are full of sugar; it's a marketing tool to suck you in to believing you're eating a healthy alternative. This is why I get frustrated with diet clubs; the treats they recommend tend to have no fat but loads of sugar, which means the weight loss is solely focused on appearance and not health and isn't a long-term solution.

Why does sugar make you fat? Sugar is a molecule that the human body does not produce and therefore is not a natural part of our metabolism. The only cells in the body that can make use of it are liver cells – these cells turn the sugar that we eat into fat (so not a very productive use). This fat is then distributed around the body. Therefore, because our bodies have no use for sugar, the more sugar you eat, the more fat is produced by the liver.

2 EAT LESS BAD FAT AND MORE GOOD FAT
Put your hand up if you're scared of the word FAT!

We usually associate it with being overweight, but it's actually an important source of energy found in food.

Fat is made up of amino acids, which are either saturated, polyunsaturated or monounsaturated, depending on their chemical structure. Some of these amino acids are essential to the human body and others are actually quite damaging to our health. This is why some fats are referred to as GOOD fats and some are labelled as BAD fats.

A really important point to remember is that regardless of whether fat is 'good' or 'bad', both provide the same number of calories (1g = 9kcal). So too much of any type of fat can eventually lead to weight gain, something we should be mindful of even when eating 'good' fats.

So if all fats have the same calorie content, what makes a bad fat 'bad', and why should you care?

Bad fats. Croissants have become one of the UK's most popular grab-and-go breakfasts. They're convenient and easy to eat on the morning commute. The catch? Each one contains around 11g of saturated fat. If you're a woman, that's half of your recommended daily allowance! If you're a man, that's one third. All in a couple of bites you probably didn't even think about or stop to enjoy.

Other foods high in saturated fat are butter, cheese, cakes, biscuits, fried food, fatty cuts of beef, lamb, pork and poultry skin. Too much of any of these can cause health problems such as high cholesterol, which, if not treated, leads to more serious illnesses like heart disease or stroke.

By swapping that daily croissant for yoghurt, oats and berries, or a protein pot (see page 121) you're already a step closer to finding a healthy balance.

Also, remember what I said about being distracted by the latest trends? Well coconut oil, for example, despite having many good properties, is very high in saturated fat and should be used moderately when cooking, just like all other oils, until research is more advanced.

Good fats. On a more positive note, unsaturated fats like monounsaturated and polyunsaturated help us to maintain a healthy cholesterol level. Monounsaturated fats are found in vegetable oils such as olive and rapeseed oil, nuts and avocados. Polyunsaturated fats are found in oily fish such as salmon, mackerel, tuna, sardines, trout and whitebait, as well as flaxseed, walnuts, chia seeds, linseed oil and sunflower oil. They also contain essential fatty acids such as omega 3.

However, it's worth mentioning again that just because these are healthy fats doesn't mean you should put away a whole grab bag of nuts a day or eat an avocado at breakfast, lunch and at dinner. They are still fats, and can still cause weight gain, so they should be eaten regularly but in moderate amounts.

You'll notice these fats featuring in a lot of my recipes, so you can feel confident that you're going to be consuming the right amount of the right fats very soon.

3 EAT MORE AND LOSE WEIGHT

Many people who hate exercising but want to lose weight follow some sort of 'starvation diet'. I can't stress enough how unhealthy this is. Your body is going to become weak and you're going to feel lethargic, dizzy and sometimes anxious. You'll also lose muscle mass and become 'flabby'.

When the body is put under this sort of starvation stress it produces the hormones cortisol and glucagon. They send signals to your liver, encouraging the retention of fat. By eating very little the body stores whatever calories it can find from the little food you are eating. So, for example, if all you have eaten all day is a bacon sandwich, your body is going to keep every calorie from that sandwich to sustain your energy levels. If you are someone who loves junk food but thinks it's okay because you only have one or two meals a day, think again. Your body is retaining all the saturated fat from that food. This way of living can eventually cause serious long-term health problems.

Eating like this slows down the metabolism, causes muscle loss and has other side effects such as bad skin, bad breath and hair loss. It's also proven to cause cellulite, fat around your liver, heart disease and depression. Now if that's not enough to convince you to eat regularly, I don't know what is!

Three meals a day. I advise everyone to enjoy three delicious and filling meals a day to keep your body's metabolic rate consistent and help you get all the right vitamins, minerals, fats and proteins your body requires.

Snacking is not a necessity unless you have huge gaps in between meals or you've got a hard workout scheduled. Some people obsess over snacking, when personally I think it's usually done out of boredom or fear of hunger. I know I sniff around the fridge if I have nothing else to do!

Regardless of what you're snacking on, it means you're continuously consuming calories that will then be stored as fat if they're not needed as fuel.

One of two exceptions where I think snacking is fine is if there's more than 5 hours between meals, just to ensure your blood sugar levels stay stable and your energy levels don't drop. The second option is pre- and post-workout. I've included some simple snack options for those days when your body will require a little more fuel.

Otherwise, NO SNACKING. If you are a serial snacker, the changes you are making could make your tummy rumble but your body will quickly get used to it.

Don't starve: eat more. Once you start consuming the right proteins, plants, grains and fats in your diet, you'll be amazed by how much you can eat (and how delicious it is) on your weight-loss journey and how good it makes you look and feel. This book contains lots of refined sugar-free recipes ideal for healthy sustainable weight loss as well as exercises that will burn calories fast.

LOSING WEIGHT IS A MIND GAME. CHANGE YOUR MIND, CHANGE YOUR BODY.

FITNESS

HIIT COMBINED WITH BODYWEIGHT EXERCISES

The human body burns calories every day regardless of the amount of exercise we do, but if you're eating more calories than your body needs, the calories turn into fat that's stored around the body.

It may seem obvious, but it's worth reiterating: when you exercise regularly (and by regularly, I mean around 3 hours a week) your body gets the extra energy it needs from calories – calories are your fuel. So it makes sense that the more exercise you do, the more calories are burnt, the more body fat is reduced.

As a side note, this doesn't mean you go and eat as many calories as you like from whatever food you fancy when you've had a great workout. We need to consider the quality of those calories. For example, there are 89 calories in a banana and about 75 calories in two pieces of chocolate, but because the chocolate has such high levels of added sugar and saturated fat, it's nowhere near as good for you as the higher calorie banana that also contains fibre and potassium.

Look at the whole picture, not just the number of calories in the food you're eating, to work out how wholesome and nourishing something is.

WEEKLY SAMPLE FITNESS PLAN

Regardless or whether you're a fitness beginner, you're intermediate or you're already very fit (advanced), if you want to lose weight, aim to exercise 4–5 times a week for 45–60 minutes at a time, choosing the rest days that best suit you.

MONDAY	Beginner, Intermediate or Advanced HIIT Workout (page 94) followed by 3 sets of 5 different bodyweight weight-loss exercises for Beginner, Intermediate or Advanced (page 56–59) OR choose a high-intensity class like boxing, spinning or circuits
TUESDAY	Beginner, Intermediate or Advanced HIIT Workout (page 94) followed by 3 sets of 5 different bodyweight weight-loss exercises for Beginner, Intermediate or Advanced (page 56–59) OR choose a high-intensity class like boxing, spinning or circuits
WEDNESDAY	REST
THURSDAY	Beginner, Intermediate or Advanced HIIT Workout (page 94) followed by 3 sets of 5 different bodyweight weight-loss exercises for Beginner, Intermediate or Advanced (page 56–59) OR choose a high-intensity class like boxing, spinning or circuits
FRIDAY	Beginner, Intermediate or Advanced HIIT Workout (page 94) followed by 3 sets of 5 different bodyweight weight-loss exercises for Beginner, Intermediate or Advanced (page 56–59) OR choose a high-intensity class like boxing, spinning or circuits
SATURDAY	REST
SUNDAY	REST

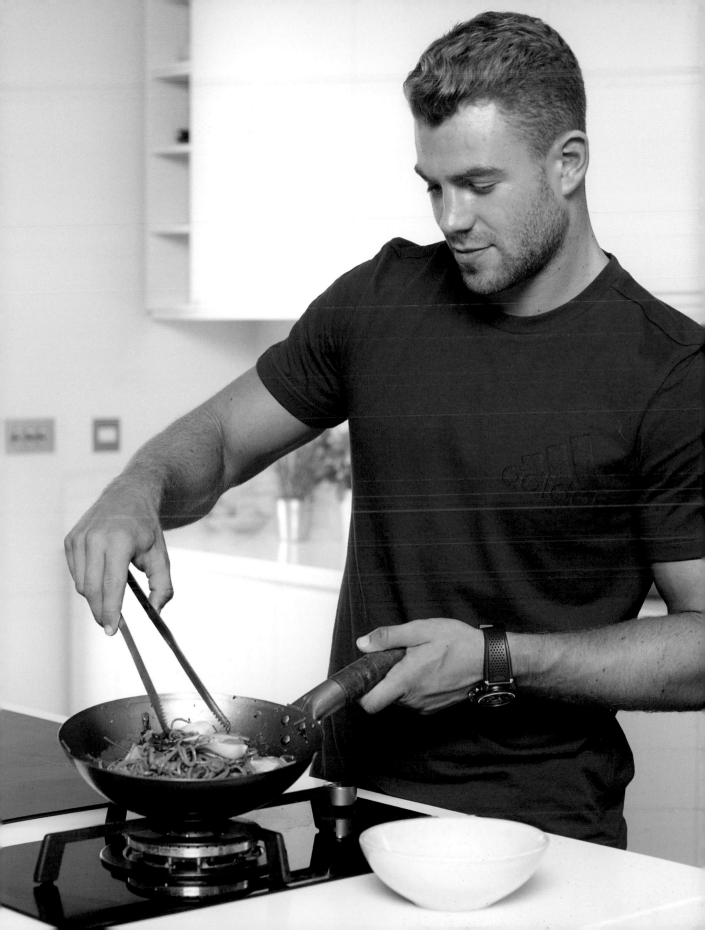

2 TONING WITHOUT BULKING AND GETTING STRONG

Strong not Skinny has become a popular mantra in the last year or so and for good reason. It's a positive sign of our more health-conscious times that a lot of women are seeking a stronger, more toned body shape, rather than fetishising the unhealthy 'skinny' look. I'm going to explain how to achieve a body that's toned or 'lean'. It's easier than you think, but some people have the wrong idea.

IS TONING JUST FOR WOMEN?

Toning is an increase of muscle tissue combined with a decrease in body fat. When people say they want to be more 'ripped', 'sculpted' or 'lean', they essentially mean toned – all of these words mean the same thing. 'Toning' has simply been more associated with women when actually it can be applied to both genders.

THE SOLUTION
FOOD

1 EAT PROTEIN

Protein is an essential part of our diets because protein is what our muscles, skin, nails and hair are made up of. Without protein, it would be impossible for us to build, repair or maintain muscle. The best way to get your protein hit if you want to get 'toned' is by eating meat low in saturated fat such as chicken (the more saturated the fat, the harder you have to work at the gym to counteract the effect of the fat), fish, seafood, eggs, beans, pulses, tofu and soy. Examples of protein with higher levels of saturated fat are lamb, beef, bacon, sausages and cheese. I'm not suggesting you completely eliminate these from your fridge – they are delicious after all! – but definitely be conscious of how often you're eating them. My advice would be to enjoy them once or twice a week.

Protein shakes. High-quality protein shakes are an easy way of introducing additional protein into your diet. Protein shakes are great for vegetarians or vegans whose diets might be low in protein or for anyone looking to continuously increase their muscle mass.

I wouldn't use protein shakes when they're high in sugar. They'll ultimately hold you back from reaching your toning or weight-loss goals. Instead use a good-quality brand recommended by trusted athletes or fitness experts.

Skin, hair and nails. You've probably seen the words collagen, keratin and elastin on shampoos, face creams in magazines and on the TV. Let me let you into a secret: they are all just proteins naturally found in our hair, skin and nails. As we get older they break down, so eating protein doesn't just help with muscle repair and growth, it affects how we look on the outside too.

2 DON'T FEAR CARBS

Protein is important, but carbohydrates are just as vital, so long as they're the right ones. If you're working out, you need complex carbs (not white processed ones!) such as brown rice, whole grains, sweet potato or quinoa with every meal to restore energy and keep your blood sugar levels balanced. The fibre and nutrients will keep cravings at bay and slow down digestion, keeping your energy levels nice and stable, and stopping you feeling hungry for longer.

FITNESS

FAT-BURNING BODYWEIGHT EXERCISES COMBINED WITH WEIGHT TRAINING

You can increase the size of your muscles through different types of weight training and eating protein, however you won't get definition without additional fat-burning exercises. Many people (mainly women) are scared of using weights because they're worried they might 'bulk' up and many people (mainly guys) think that by using just weights they will gain LEAN muscle (that's muscle not surrounded by fat). Both of these assumptions are wrong. Women CAN use weights without bulking, and men MUST combine weight training with fat-burning cardio if they want to appear toned.

So, what you need to do to become TONED is:

- Lose the fat that's covering your muscles (I should mention here that if you're already very overweight, it's a good idea to make weight loss your first goal and start off on page 24, then once you've arrived at a healthy weight, make your way here).

- Build more muscle.

- Combine the two for sustainable results.

My style of weight training combined with fat-burning bodyweight exercises for toning will help you build muscle and increase the rate at which you burn calories simply by doing nothing at all (this is your resting metabolic rate), so you lose fat faster.

WEEKLY SAMPLE FITNESS PLAN

Regardless or whether you're a fitness beginner, you're intermediate or you're already very fit (advanced), if you want to tone, aim to exercise 4–5 times a week for 30–45 minutes, choosing the rest days that best suit you.

Advanced A session can be swapped for classes such as yoga, Pilates or body pump.

	BEGINNER
MONDAY	3 sets of 5–10 different bodyweight weight-loss, toning and core exercises (pages 56–69) such as Burpees, Explosive Jumping Jacks, Jumping Lunges, Blast Offs, Planks and V Sit-Ups
TUESDAY	3 sets of 5–10 different bodyweight weight-loss, toning and core exercises (pages 56–69) such as Bear Crawls, High Knees, Jumping Squats, Planks with Shoulder Taps, Toe-Touch Planks and Elbow to Knee Crunches
WEDNESDAY	REST
THURSDAY	3 sets of 5–10 different bodyweight weight-loss, toning and core exercises (pages 56–69) such as Burpees, Bear Crawls, Resistant Band Walks, Mountain Climbers, Jumping Squats and Blast Offs
FRIDAY	REST
SATURDAY	3 sets of 5–10 different bodyweight weight-loss, toning and core exercises (pages 56–69) such as Explosive Jumping Jacks, Elbow to Knee Crunches, Resistant Band Walks, Planks, V Sit-Ups and Toe-Touch Planks
SUNDAY	REST

INTERMEDIATE	ADVANCED
3 sets of 5 different bodyweight weight-loss, toning, core and TRX exercises (pages 56–73) such as Burpees, Jumping Squats, Planks, Runners' Lunges and Bicep Curls THEN 5 weight-training exercises (pages 74–91) focusing on 1–2 muscle groups every day, such as Quads and Glutes, and Hamstrings	3 sets of 5 different bodyweight weight-loss, toning, core and TRX exercises (pages 56–73) such as Burpees, Jumping Squats, Planks, Runners' Lunges and Bicep Curls THEN 5 weight-training exercises (pages 74–91) focusing on 1–2 muscle groups every day, such as Quads and Glutes, and Hamstrings
3 sets of 5 different bodyweight weight-loss, toning, core and TRX exercises (pages 56–73) such as Explosive Jumping Jacks, Jumping Lunges, Toe-Touch Planks, Knee Tucks and Pikes THEN 5 weight-training exercises (pages 74–91) focusing on 1–2 muscle groups every day, such as Back and Biceps	45-minute yoga class
REST	REST
3 sets of 5 different bodyweight weight-loss, toning, core and TRX exercises (pages 56–73) such as Bear Crawls, Blast Offs, Planks, V Sit Ups and Runners' Lunges THEN 5 weight-training exercises (pages 74–91) focusing on 1–2 muscle groups every day, such as Chest and Triceps	3 sets of 5 different bodyweight weight-loss, toning, core and TRX exercises (pages 56–73) such as Explosive Jumping Jacks, Jumping Lunges, Toe-Touch Planks, Knee Tucks and Pikes THEN 5 weight-training exercises (pages 74–91) focusing on 1–2 muscle groups every day, such as Back and Biceps
REST	45-minute Pilates class
3 sets of 5 different bodyweight weight-loss, toning, core and TRX exercises (pages 56–73) such as High Knees, Resistant Band Walks, Mountain Climbers and Bicep Curls THEN 5 weight-training exercises (pages 74–91) focusing on 1–2 muscle groups every day, such as Shoulders, and Quads and Glutes	3 sets of 5 different bodyweight weight-loss, toning, core and TRX exercises (pages 56–73) such as Bear Crawls, Blast Offs, Planks, V Sit-Ups and Runners' Lunges THEN 5 weight- training exercises (page 74–91) focusing on 1–2 muscle groups every day, such as Chest and Triceps
REST	REST

3 HEALTHY WEIGHT GAIN THROUGH LEAN MUSCLE

If you want to put on weight the healthy way, by nourishing your body with wholesome meals to gain lean muscle, then this book is perfect for you. Maybe you're underweight and lacking energy and you've made the decision to change that, or perhaps you're already a healthy weight but would prefer to be bigger. Either way, it is important that you don't feel the only way to do this is by eating food high in saturated fat and sugar while sitting on the sofa!

THE SOLUTION
FOOD

1 BE MINDFUL

I've seen plenty of influential people posting pictures with spreads of chocolate, sweets, popcorn, crisps and fizzy drinks on social media saying they're 'gaining' or trying to put on weight. This message is so damaging and misleading for followers. I'm all for a cheat meal and the odd treat, but using junk food to gain weight is not the right way to go about it. Regardless of what your goal is, bingeing on food full of sugar and saturated fat is harmful (see page 24–26). Just because you can 'afford' to gain weight, it doesn't mean you can afford to have mood swings, headaches and high cholesterol. Gaining weight requires you to be just as mindful of what you're eating as someone losing weight or toning.

2 EAT LITTLE AND OFTEN

Healthy weight gain usually means eating more food than you're used to, but if you can't stomach three bigger meals a day with the odd snack, then try changing the pattern of your eating. Having smaller, more frequent meals throughout the day may work better for you and your lifestyle. A good idea is to prepare your smaller meals the night before, then you'll feel organised and be less likely to skip eating as it's ready to go.

Again, just like any other goal, meals should be balanced and nutritious, containing lean protein, complex carbs, good fats and plants. A great snack would be apple slices with nut butter or carrots with houmous.

Get those healthy fats and vitamins inside you!

FITNESS

HIIT COMBINED WITH BODYWEIGHT, TRX OR WEIGHT-TRAINING EXERCISES

A note on bodyweight exercises. If your goal is to gain weight through lean muscle, then not only will you have to eat more of the right food, you'll also need to work out more. Exercise burns calories but it also helps build muscle. So don't fear the calorie-burning element of training; as long as you are eating enough to restore the calories lost, you won't lose more weight.

When you're starting out, bodyweight exercises are the most suitable style of exercise for gaining weight healthily. Using your body to build strength in your muscles is effective without being too strenuous – you could also use resistance bands and very light weights. What's great about all of this is that everything can be done at home – ideal for anyone not quite ready to face the gym.

Pilates and yoga. Low-intensity exercise like Pilates and yoga is amazing at improving balance, strength and core stability. They are essentially a form of bodyweight exercises as you have to balance and perform certain moves for short periods of time. However, they also offer the benefits of stretching, mobilising and a sense of relaxation.

WEEKLY SAMPLE FITNESS PLAN

Regardless or whether you're a fitness beginner, you're intermediate or you're already very fit (advanced), if you want to tone, aim to exercise 4–5 times a week for 45–60 minutes, choosing the rest days that best suit you.

Advanced A session can be swapped for classes such as boxing, body pump or HIIT circuits.

	BEGINNER
MONDAY	Beginner HIIT Workout (page 94) followed by 3 sets of 5 different bodyweight toning exercises (pages 60–65) or weight-training exercises (pages 74–91). Weight- training exercises should focus on 1–2 different muscle groups each day
TUESDAY	Beginner HIIT Workout (page 94) followed by 3 sets of 5 different bodyweight toning exercises (pages 60–65) or weight-training exercises (pages 74–91). Weight- training exercises should focus on 1–2 different muscle groups each day
WEDNESDAY	REST
THURSDAY	Beginner HIIT Workout (page 94) followed by 3 sets of 5 different bodyweight toning exercises (pages 60–65) or weight-training exercises (pages 74–91). Weight- training exercises should focus on 1–2 different muscle groups each day
FRIDAY	REST
SATURDAY	Beginner HIIT Workout (page 94) followed by 3 sets of 5 different bodyweight toning exercises (pages 60–65) or weight-training exercises (pages 74–91). Weight- training exercises should focus on 1–2 different muscle groups each day
SUNDAY	REST

INTERMEDIATE	ADVANCED
Intermediate HIIT Workout (page 94) followed by 3 sets of 5 different bodyweight toning exercises (pages 60–65) or TRX (pages 70–73) or weight-training exercises (pages 74–91). Weight-training exercises should focus on 1–2 different muscle groups each day	Advanced HIIT Workout (page 94) followed by 3 sets of 5 different TRX (pages 70–73) or weight-training exercises (pages 74–91). Weight-training exercises should focus on 1–2 different muscle groups each day
Intermediate HIIT Workout (page 94) followed by 3 sets of 5 different bodyweight toning exercises (pages 60–65) or TRX (pages 70–73) or weight-training exercises (pages 74–91). Weight-training exercises should focus on 1–2 different muscle groups each day	1-hour boxing class
REST	REST
Intermediate HIIT Workout (page 94) followed by 3 sets of 5 different bodyweight toning exercises (pages 60–65) or TRX (pages 70–73) or weight-training exercises (pages 74–91). Weight-training exercises should focus on 1–2 different muscle groups each day	Advanced HIIT Workout (page 94) followed by 3 sets of 5 different TRX (pages 70–73) or weight-training exercises (pages 74–91). Weight-training exercises should focus on 1–2 different muscle groups each day
REST	45 minutes HIIT circuits (page 93)
Intermediate HIIT Workout (page 94) followed by 3 sets of 5 different bodyweight toning exercises (pages 60–65) or TRX (pages 70–73) or weight-training exercises (pages 74–91). Weight-training exercises should focus on 1–2 different muscle groups each day	Advanced HIIT Workout (page 94) followed by 3 sets of 5 different TRX (pages 70–73) or weight-training exercises (pages 74–91). Weight-training exercises should focus on 1–2 different muscle groups each day
REST	REST

4 YOUR MENTAL HEALTH AND INCREASED ENERGY LEVELS

I believe that how you look has a huge impact on how you feel and how you think. But is appearance the most important thing?

The BIGGEST and BEST improvements I see in all of my clients is their mentality and energy levels and, in the grand scheme of things, these are the most important and gratifying improvements of all.

When I suffered from my injuries, stopping exercise and eating what I wanted made me lose confidence in my profession and that became my wake-up call. At that time, it was my emotional state that became the real catalyst for change, much more than how I looked.

THE MIND IS A POWERFUL THING

I wonder how many people can, hand on heart say, 'I'm happy with the way I feel and think about myself'?

If you often feel tired, lethargic, anxious, down, insecure, weak or your body suffers from aches and pains, then you may not be happy and this needs to change.

Our mind is so powerful, it tells us what to do, how to feel and how to act every second of every day. Yet, we often forget about this when it comes to nourishment and exercise. The mind is who we are; nevertheless it can be controlled and nurtured through long-term healthy living.

THE SOLUTION

1 TACKLE GUILT-MAKING CRAVINGS

Cravings usually make us feel bad when we succumb to them; after all, it isn't often that we crave lettuce or broccoli! Cravings tend to crop up when we're either lacking some essential nutrient our bodies need, or when we subconsciously seek a 'feeling' that food gives us. For example, chocolate contains phenylethylamine, which triggers a release of endorphins – endorphins are hormones that result in a sense of relaxation. That's why chocolate is seen as a comfort food. But there are other ways to release these endorphins into the body – exercise being one.

We also trigger cravings when we booze. Alcohol makes us dehydrated and causes our bodies to lose salt and electrolytes that we need to replace. This, together with our need for energy and comfort, results in 'junk food' cravings. If you're planning a big night out, make sure your fridge is stocked with healthy alternatives to the usual 'morning-after-the-night-before' fry up, containing moderate levels of sodium and carbs to combat those cravings, such as Parma ham, feta cheese, halloumi, olives, trimmed bacon, lean sausages or minced meat. I wouldn't recommend eating these regularly, but they definitely hit the spot the next morning (or afternoon!).

But it doesn't matter how much willpower you have, you will be faced with hurdles. Nobody's perfect, we're all human and we all experience temptations and cravings. My advice would be: if your craving for something unhealthy lasts a few days and the alternatives haven't worked, then enjoy and savour a small portion of it and move on. Always put up a good fight as more than likely you're simply fighting an addiction to something.

JUNK FOOD YOU'VE CRAVED FOR AN HOUR? OR THE BODY YOU'VE CRAVED FOR A LIFETIME?

2 GET YOUR NEAREST AND DEAREST ON BOARD

You can't convince everyone, believe me I've tried. However, if you have the urge to get up and get healthy (which you must do, since you're reading this!) then try and get your friends and family on board too.

Be a leader, be the instigator and encourage those around you to join your journey so you can all support and motivate each other. I always say start by focusing on yourself. This still holds true, but having someone close to share your experience with is definitely a huge advantage. They'll only thank you for it – my sister thanks me all the time!

3 FIND NEW WAYS OF SOCIALISING

If your current unhealthy lifestyle is affecting the way you feel and act, this will likely be affecting everyone else around you. But they aren't reacting to your natural personality, the person you are at your healthiest, and this is nothing that can't be fixed through delicious food and exercise. If on the other hand you're worried how adopting a new healthier lifestyle is going to affect your social life, then don't panic. I'm going to show you how to make fitness and eating well a major and enjoyable part of your social life.

I often work in Central London and I was surprised by the amount of midweek drinking that goes on after work. If you drink during the week and then again on the weekends, it's worth reconsidering your lifestyle. If drinking with clients or colleagues is essential, I'd suggest you find new ways of socialising at the weekends. Alcohol will delay you on your health and fitness journey no matter what your goal is.

Before you call me a boring 23-year-old, I do like to go out with my mates, but alcohol doesn't always have to be a big part of the evening for us to have fun. Alcohol is toxic and if drunk regularly (10–14 units a week) it can cause long-term health problems such as liver disease, brain damage, vitamin deficiencies and immune system dysfunction. And if long-term health problems don't scare you, then what about the uncontrollable cravings for greasy food for the next couple of days?

Here's what you can do instead:

- Find new and exciting restaurants that offer healthy options.

- Catch up on a walk rather than over a drink.

- Play football, netball, golf, tennis or any kind of sport together.

- Shopping – treat yourself to new gym clothes.

- Nights in filled with delicious food (see my Social Sharer recipes on page 172).

- Try the theatre, cinema, museums etc.

It was refreshing to hear that in 2016 the UK spent more on health and fitness than they did on alcohol as a result of gym memberships increasing by a staggering 44 percent. Hopefully this continues and Britain becomes better known for healthy living rather than binge drinking.

4 CONQUER SHYNESS AND EMBARRASSMENT AT THE GYM

Clearly more and more people are jumping on the fitness thing, so when you go to the gym or fitness class, why do you feel shy or embarrassed? Of course everyone is at different fitness and experience levels, but we all have to start somewhere.

Not only will you gain confidence from being at the gym and taking part in fitness classes, but you'll start making new friends if you're consistent with your classes.

Fitness is there to be enjoyed by everyone and if you can make friends doing it, then BONUS!

5 EAT OUT BUT EAT WELL

I love a good restaurant and I love eating out (mainly because I hate washing up!)

If you spend a large portion of your salary on eating out (including lunch at work), then just make sure you're being mindful with your food choices. What is worth remembering is that if you make your own lunch (whether it's the day before or in the office canteen) you know exactly what you've put in there, and you can keep track of your calories. Making your own meals more often also means that those times when you do eat out become a lot more exciting and feel like a real treat.

I decided to reduce how often I ate out at restaurants and instead buy fresh ingredients and cook my lunch at home. It means sometimes waiting a little longer or eating a little earlier than I would ideally like to, but that's fine. The pros – knowing that what I am eating isn't cooked with added sugar and tonnes of butter or with poor quality ingredients – way outweigh the cons.

When you do go out to restaurants, lots of them now offer delicious and healthy alternatives or they have a side menu longer than your arm, so you can always swap creamy mash potato for sweet potato wedges. But if you want to indulge in creamy mash every now and again, GO FOR IT. Eating out is a treat and should feel like it.

Follow my tips for when you go to restaurants with friends so you don't blow all your hard work, but still enjoy yourself:

- Read the menu online and decide on a couple of choices before you get there.

- Never go to a restaurant starving – you'll order and eat way more than you need to.

- Stick to cuisines you know offer healthier meal choices e.g. Japanese, Thai or steakhouses.

- Decide on how many alcoholic drinks you're going to have beforehand and stick to it.

- Choose a starter over a pudding.

REMEMBER: I'm not saying don't ever enjoy eating at a restaurant again, but if you are doing it all the time and you're not finding the balance between dining out and eating healthily, you won't reach your goal.

6 MAKE FITNESS PART OF YOUR DAILY ROUTINE

There are small changes you can make in everyday life that can make you feel more energised and healthy:

- Get off the bus or train one stop early and walk the rest of the journey.

- Sacrifice 30 minutes of TV for 30 minutes of exercise – there is always catch up!

- Squat or lunge while brushing your teeth or waiting for the kettle to boil.

- Walk to school with the kids so the whole family gets to stretch their legs.

- Instead of lazy Sundays have leisurely Sundays, like walks around the park.

With just small changes like these, your body gets a little fitter every day. Happy hormones are released and you become a lot more energised.

Everyone is different, so what relaxes and calms one person doesn't necessarily work for someone else. I love to box to let off steam, but I understand this isn't everyone's cup of tea. Instead have a look at the table overleaf for some inspiration.

WEEKLY SAMPLE FITNESS PLAN

Beginner Try incorporating 3 feel-good 45–60 minute exercises into your routine a week like beginner's yoga, Pilates or water aerobics. You could also go for long walks in local parks during lunch breaks or to start your day – just keep the pace up slightly.

Intermediate Aim to do 4 feel-good 45–60 minute exercises a week. Hiking in the outdoors can be quite relaxing, especially if you enjoy nature.

Advanced Incorporate 5 feel-good 45–60 minute exercises into your routine per week, like yoga, Pilates or swimming or you could go for long walks, hikes, cycling alone or with the family on weekends.

	BEGINNER
MONDAY	1.5 mile walk to work 1 hour beginner's yoga class
TUESDAY	1.5 mile walk to work
WEDNESDAY	1.5 mile walk in local park during lunch break 45 minute beginner's Pilates class
THURSDAY	REST
FRIDAY	1.5 mile walk to work
SATURDAY	REST
SUNDAY	1 hour swim

INTERMEDIATE	ADVANCED
1.5 mile walk to work 1 hour intermediate yoga class	1.5 mile walk to work 1 hour intermediate yoga class
1.5 mile walk in local park during lunch break 45 minute intermediate Pilates class	1.5 mile walk in local park during lunch break 1 hour intermediate Pilates class
1.5 mile walk to work	1.5 mile walk to work
1.5 mile walk in local park during lunch break 45–60 minute intermediate high-intensity water workout	1.5 mile walk in local park during lunch break 1 hour intermediate high-intensity water workout
1.5 mile walk to work	1.5 mile walk to work 1 hour intermediate yoga class
1 hour hike in the woods or park	1 hour hike in the woods or park
REST	1 hour cycle

WEEKLY SAMPLE FITNESS PLAN

Core strength should be included with every workout regardless of your goal. But if you're looking to work solely on your core, try incorporating the following exercises into your weekly fitness routine, depending on your fitness and experience levels.

Beginner Try 3 sets of 5 bodyweight core exercises 3 times a week. Your workouts should last approximately 20 minutes.

Intermediate Aim to do 3 sets of 5 bodyweight core exercises and 3 sets of 3 TRX exercises 3 times a week. Each session should last approximately 30 minutes. Some gyms offer TRX-specific classes, so keep an eye out if you're interested in trying them.

Advanced Incorporate 3 sets of 5 bodyweight core exercises and 3 sets of 3 TRX exercises into your weekly routine 4–5 times a week. Your sessions should last approximately 30 minutes. Some gyms offer TRX-specific classes, so keep an eye out if you're interested in trying them..

	BEGINNER
MONDAY	3 sets of 5 different bodyweight core exercises (pages 64–69) such as Planks, Toe-Touch Planks, V Sit-Ups, Elbow to Knee Crunches and Mountain Climbers
TUESDAY	REST
WEDNESDAY	3 sets of 5 different bodyweight core exercises (pages 64–69) such as Planks, Toe-Touch Planks, V Sit-Ups, Elbow to Knee Crunches and Mountain Climbers
THURSDAY	REST
FRIDAY	3 sets of 5 different bodyweight core exercises (pages 64–69) such as Planks, Toe-Touch Planks, V Sit-Ups, Elbow to Knee Crunches and Mountain Climbers
SATURDAY	REST
SUNDAY	REST

INTERMEDIATE	ADVANCED
3 sets of 5 different bodyweight core exercises (pages 64–69) such as Planks, Toe-Touch planks, V Sit-Ups, Elbow to Knee Crunches and Mountain Climbers AND 3 sets of 3 different TRX exercises (pages 70–73) such as Pistol Squats, Runners' Lunges and Bicep Curls	3 sets of 5 different bodyweight core exercises (pages 64–69) such as Planks, Toe-Touch Planks, V Sit-Ups, Elbow to Knee Crunches and Mountain Climbers AND 3 sets of 3 different TRX exercises (pages 70–73) such as Pistol Squats, Runners' Lunges and Bicep Curls
REST	3 sets of 5 different bodyweight core exercises (pages 64–69) such as Planks, Toe-Touch Planks, V Sit-Ups, Elbow to Knee Crunches and Mountain Climbers AND 3 sets of 3 different TRX exercises (pages 70–73) such as Runners' Lunges, Bicep Curls and Knee Tucks
3 sets of 5 different bodyweight core exercises (pages 64–69) such as Plank, Toe-Touch plank, V Sit-Ups, Elbow to Knee Crunches and Mountain Climbers AND 3 sets of 3 different TRX exercises (pages 70–73) such as Knee Tucks, Pikes and Pistol Squats	3 sets of 5 different bodyweight core exercises (pages 64–69) such as Planks, Toe-Touch Planks, V Sit-Ups, Elbow to Knee Crunches and Mountain Climbers AND 3 sets of 3 different TRX exercises (pages 70–73) such as Knee Tucks, Pikes and Pistol Squats
REST	REST
3 sets of 5 different bodyweight core exercises (pages 64–69) such as Plank, Toe-Touch plank, V Sit-Ups, Elbow to Knee Crunches and Mountain Climbers AND 3 sets of 3 different TRX exercises (pages 70–73) such as Runners' Lunges, Bicep Curls and Knee Tucks	3 sets of 5 different bodyweight core exercises (pages 64–69) such as Planks, Toe-Touch Planks, V Sit-Ups, Elbow to Knee Crunches and Mountain Climbers AND 3 sets of 3 different TRX exercises (pages 70–73) such as Runners' Lunges, Pikes and Knee Tucks
REST	3 sets of 5 different bodyweight core exercises (pages 64–69) such as Planks, Toe-Touch Planks, V Sit-Ups, Elbow to Knee Crunches and Mountain Climbers AND 3 sets of 3 different TRX exercises (pages 70–73) such as Bicep Curls, Pistol Squats and Knee Tucks
REST	REST

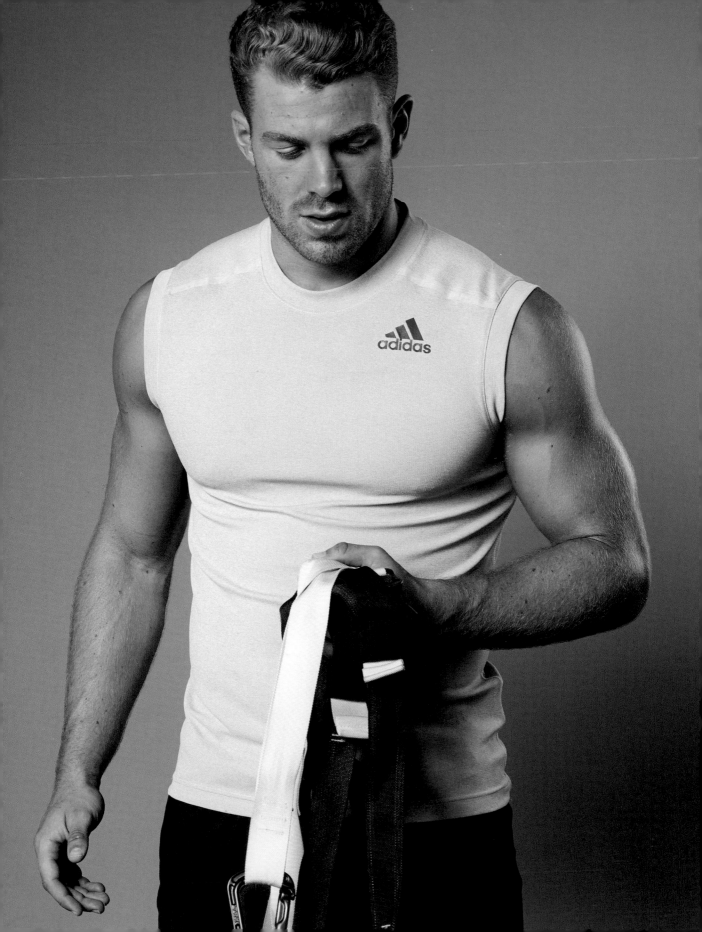

IT'S TIME

Now you know what your goal is, and exactly what you need to do to achieve it. Are you raring to go? You'd better be, because you're going to be pushing yourself hard! But I promise you that once you get into the habit of making exercise a part of your weekly routine, you'll never look back.

Now, it's time to get started!

- Draw up your personal fitness plan for the coming week based on the advice for your goal and the weekly sample fitness plans in this chapter.

- Create a personal meal plan for the week based on the food advice for your goal and using the delicious recipes in the next chapter, then go out and stock your fridge!

- Kit yourself out with the equipment you need. Unless you're looking to gain weight healthily, or you're an intermediate fitness level or above looking to tone, there's no need for weights at all. All you need is a fitness step, a resistance band and a TRX strap. Your bodyweight does the rest.

Now get ready to make that first step on a journey that will be the best thing you'll ever do for yourself, your friends and your family. I know you can do this.

YOU HAVE TO GET UP EVERY MORNING AND TELL YOURSELF, I CAN DO THIS.

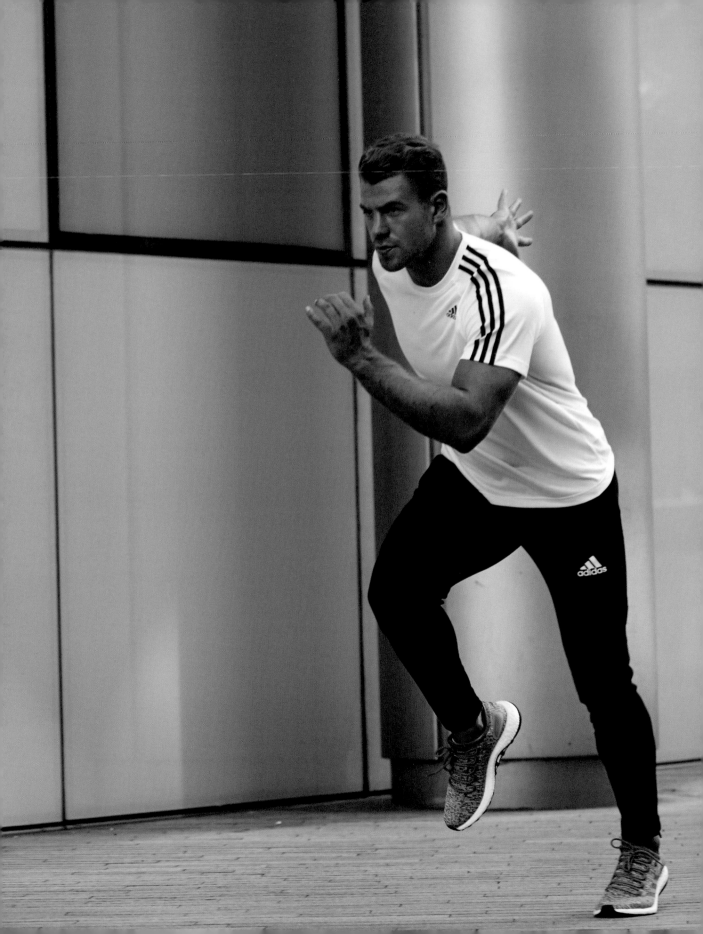

CHAPTER 2

NOW GET MOVING

ONE OF MY AIMS IS TO HELP YOU FIND YOUR FAVOURITE TYPE OF EXERCISE SO YOU CAN STAY MOTIVATED, REACH YOUR GOALS AND MAINTAIN YOUR INCREDIBLE RESULTS. IF YOU DON'T ENJOY WHAT YOU'RE DOING, WHY SHOULD YOU STICK AT IT? THAT'S WHY I'M A BIG BELIEVER IN VARIETY AND FLEXIBILITY WHEN IT COMES TO FITNESS.

MY FAVOURITE EXERCISES VARY. OBVIOUSLY I LOVE PLAYING FOOTBALL, WHICH IS A GREAT CARDIO WORKOUT, BUT ONCE I BECAME A PERSONAL TRAINER I KNEW THE BODY TYPE I WANTED TO ACHIEVE AND HOW I WANTED TO FEEL, AND THAT, PRETTY MUCH, WAS HOW I DISCOVERED MY FAVOURITE STYLES OF EXERCISE.

TO GET TO WHERE I WANTED TO BE, I NEEDED TO BUILD MUSCLE WHILE BURNING FAT. USUALLY, THAT MEANS LIFTING WEIGHTS BUT – I DON'T KNOW ABOUT YOU – THAT CAN BORE ME! SO I WORKED ON CREATING A BESPOKE TONING AND FAT-BURNING EXERCISE PLAN FOR A BIT OF VARIETY. IT WORKED SO WELL FOR ME, I USE THIS APPROACH THROUGHOUT MY DAY-TO-DAY WORK AND WITH ALL MY CLIENTS.

YOU CAN USE THIS CHAPTER AS A COMPREHENSIVE EXERCISE INDEX FOR A RANGE OF FITNESS LEVELS OR IF YOU'RE OUT OF FITNESS IDEAS AND LOOKING FOR A BIT OF INSPIRATION.

BODYWEIGHT EXERCISES

Ideal for in the gym, at home, the park or anywhere!

Please note: no equipment and very little space is required for these.

For me, this style of exercise is a game changer. This should shut down all of the excuses I hear from people who say they don't like the gym, can't afford a membership or don't have time to work out.

Bodyweight exercises are simple yet super effective for anyone trying to lose weight, and at the same time will help to improve strength and fitness levels. They are also ideal for building up core strength, the most vital area of the body (see page 45).

Any bodyweight exercise will give you results regardless of your goal, but these are my favourites. You can burn up to 300 calories in a 20–30 minute bodyweight exercise session. So get it done, no excuses.

BODYWEIGHT WEIGHT-LOSS EXERCISES

Bodyweight exercises such as burpees, jumping jacks, high knees, bear crawls and alligator crawls will quickly increase your heart rate, making your body burn calories quicker. As these exercises require you to use your strength (unlike jogging) you start to build lean muscle, which increases your metabolic rate and also helps to burn calories, even when you're resting.

BURPEES

This is an all-over body workout consisting of a squat thrust that ends in a standing position. Don't forget to engage your core (see page 45) and squeeze your glutes as you stand up.

Beginner: 20 seconds non-stop and 40 seconds rest – 3–5 sets
Intermediate: 30 seconds non-stop and 30 seconds rest – 3–5 sets
Advanced: 40 seconds non-stop and 20 seconds rest – 3–5 sets

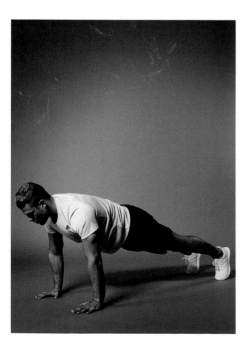 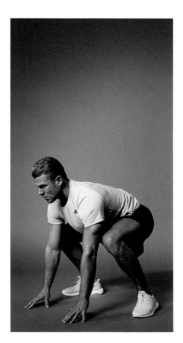 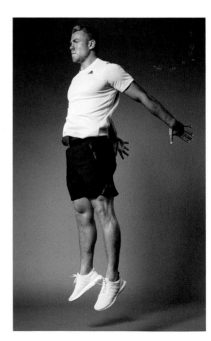

EXPLOSIVE JUMPING JACKS

Doing non-stop jumping jacks for a period of time will get the heart racing. Start by standing in a pencil position, arms by your sides, then jump into a starfish position with arms and legs outspread. Make sure you lift off the ground with power when you jump into the starfish position.

Beginner: 20 seconds non-stop and 40 seconds rest – 3–5 sets
Intermediate: 30 seconds non stop and 30 seconds rest – 3–5 sets
Advanced: 40 seconds non stop and 20 seconds rest – 3–5 sets

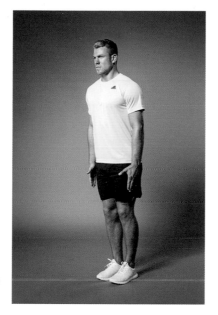 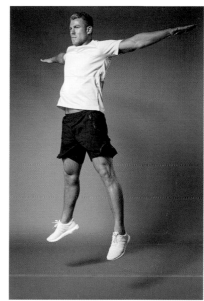

HIGH KNEES

This is another cardio-focused exercise. Simply stand on the spot and march as fast as you can, lifting your knees up to your waist.

Beginner: 20 seconds non-stop and 40 seconds rest – 3–5 sets
Intermediate: 30 seconds non-stop and 30 seconds rest – 3–5 sets
Advanced: 40 seconds non-stop and 20 seconds rest – 3–5 sets

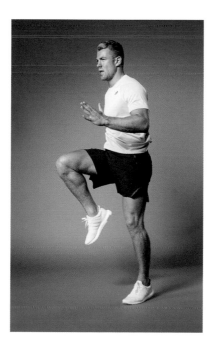 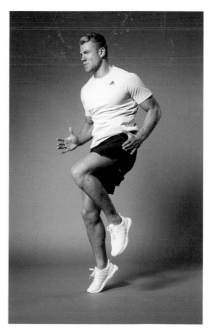

BEAR CRAWLS

Crouch on your hands and your toes, keeping your knees bent so your weight is on your toes and your knees are off the floor. Crawl forwards and backwards without letting your knees touch the ground, keeping your back straight and your bum down.

Beginner: 20 seconds non-stop and 40 seconds rest – 3–5 sets
Intermediate: 30 seconds non-stop and 30 seconds rest – 3–5 sets
Advanced: 40 seconds non-stop and 20 seconds rest – 3–5 sets

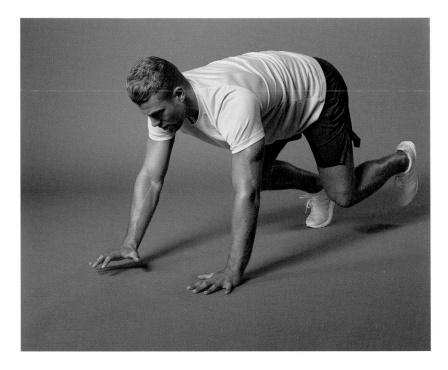

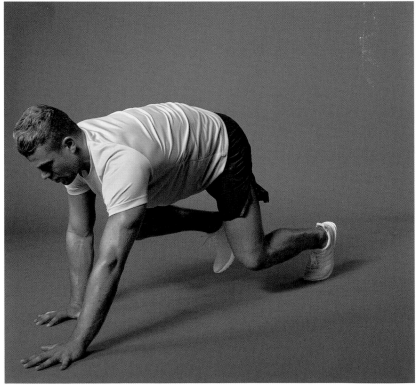

ALLIGATOR CRAWLS

A great core and arm workout. Get into a push-up position, with your feet on the floor and your arms and back straight. Then crawl forwards, engaging your core, essentially dragging your body using your arms, upper body and core muscles.

Beginner: 20 seconds non-stop and 40 seconds rest – 3–5 sets
Intermediate: 30 seconds non-stop and 30 seconds rest – 3–5 sets
Advanced: 40 seconds non-stop and 20 seconds rest – 3–5 sets

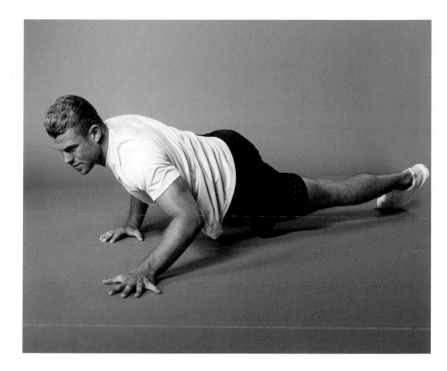

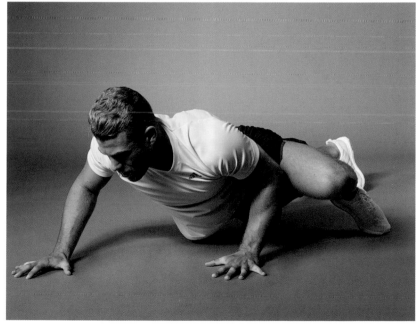

BLAST OFFS

Get into a plank position and bend your knees without touching the floor, keeping your hands in place and pushing your bum back towards your heels. 'Blast' forwards using your legs back to a plank. Repeat as quickly as you can.

Beginner: 20 seconds non-stop and 40 seconds rest – 3–5 sets
Intermediate: 30 seconds non-stop and 30 seconds rest – 3–5 sets
Advanced: 40 seconds non-stop and 20 seconds rest – 3–5 sets

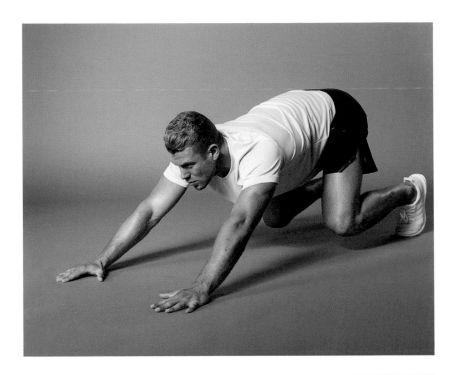

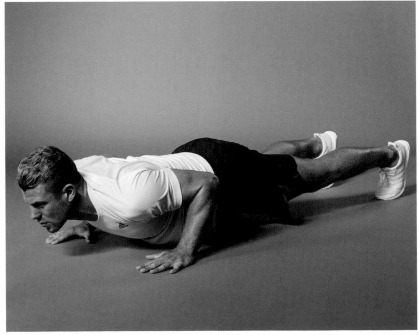

RESISTANT BAND WALKS

This does require a very small and affordable piece of equipment, but it is worth every penny as the bands can be used for leg or arm exercises. Place the band around the ankles, get into a squat position and move like a crab sideways or forwards, one foot at a time, swapping over the band. Do not come out of the squat position until it's time to rest.

Beginner: 20 seconds non-stop and 40 seconds rest – 3–5 sets
Intermediate: 30 seconds non-stop and 30 seconds rest – 3–5 sets
Advanced: 40 seconds non stop and 20 seconds rest – 3–5 sets

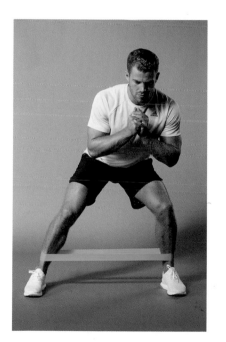

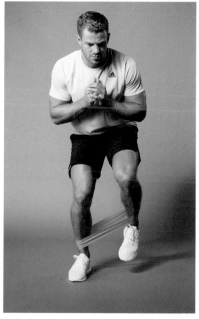

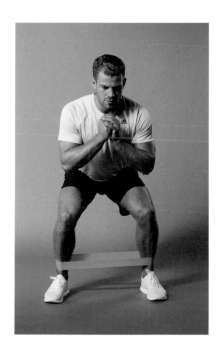

BODYWEIGHT CORE EXERCISES

Remember, your core is your body's pillar. It constantly supports you and therefore including core exercises into your weekly work out routines is ESSENTIAL for EVERYONE. Strengthening our core will help prevent injuries, back pain, poor posture, bad balance and stability. Now make sure you suck your stomach in and really engage your core muscles whilst completing these exercises.

PLANK

This is an effective core and full-body strength and conditioning exercise. Lie in a plank position, face down, leaning on your elbows and your toes. Make sure your bum is down and your core is engaged (see page 45) the whole time.

Beginner: 20 seconds non-stop and 40 seconds rest – 3–5 sets
Intermediate: 30 seconds non-stop and 30 seconds rest – 3–5 sets
Advanced: 40 seconds non-stop and 20 seconds rest – 3–5 sets

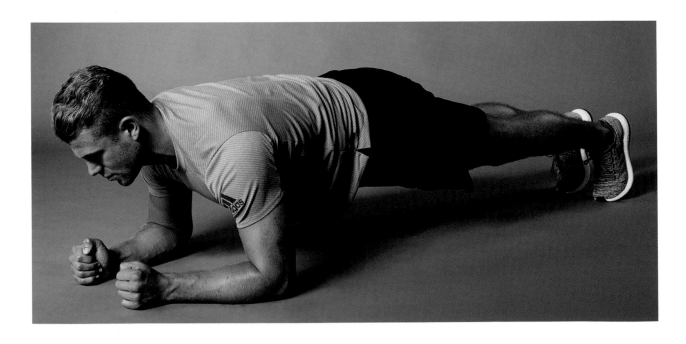

TOE-TOUCH PLANK

Get into a full plank position (on your hands, not on your elbows). Use one arm to balance and move the other arm backwards with your body to touch your toes. Alternate your arms and legs every time.

Beginner: 20 seconds non-stop and 40 seconds rest – 3–5 sets

Intermediate: 30 seconds non-stop and 30 seconds rest – 3–5 sets

Advanced: 40 seconds non-stop and 20 seconds rest – 3–5 sets

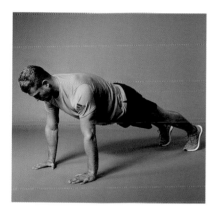
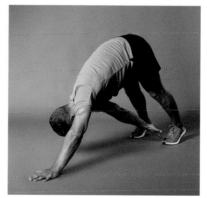
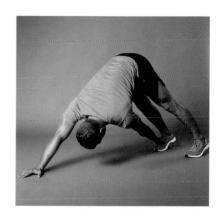

PLANK WITH SHOULDER TAPS

Get into a full plank position (see above), making sure your back is straight and your bum always stays down. Then lift alternate arms to touch the opposite shoulder with your hands.

Beginner: 20 seconds non-stop and 40 seconds rest – 3–5 sets

Intermediate: 30 seconds non-stop and 30 seconds rest – 3–5 sets

Advanced: 40 seconds non-stop and 20 seconds rest – 3–5 sets

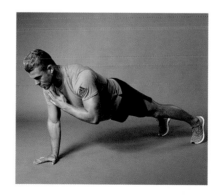
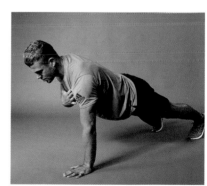

MOUNTAIN CLIMBERS

Another heart-pumping core exercise that really gets the lower core muscles working. Go on all fours, with your back straight and bum down, then bring your knees in to touch your chest as quickly as possible, alternating your legs.

Beginner: 20 seconds non-stop and 40 seconds rest – 3–5 sets

Intermediate: 30 seconds non-stop and 30 seconds rest – 3–5 sets

Advanced: 40 seconds non-stop and 20 seconds rest – 3–5 sets

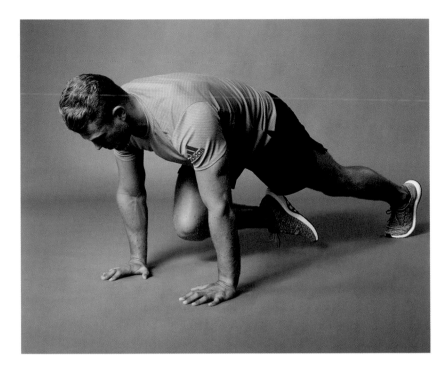

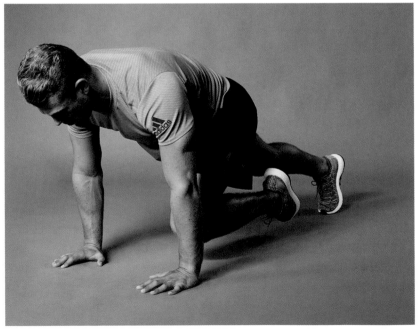

CROSS MOUNTAIN CLIMBERS

Like the standard mountain climber, this is a great exercise for working the whole abdominal area as well as the obliques and hip flexors. Go on all fours, with your back straight and bum down, ensuring your spine is in line from top to bottom. Then, alternating legs, bring one knee to the opposite elbow as quickly as you can.

Beginner: 20 seconds non-stop and 40 seconds rest – 3–5 sets
Intermediate: 30 seconds non-stop and 30 seconds rest – 3–5 sets
Advanced: 40 seconds non-stop and 20 seconds rest – 3–5 sets

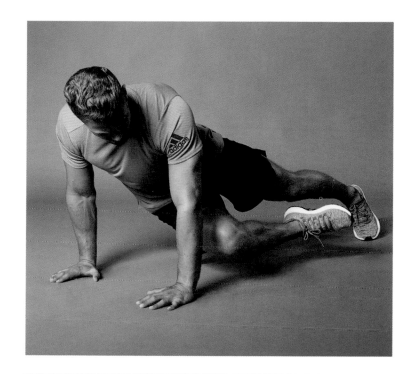

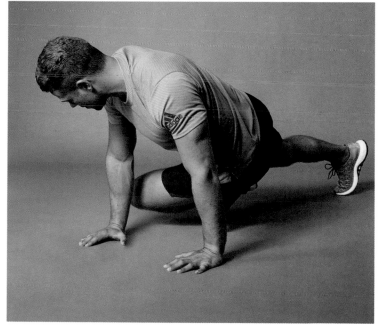

V SIT-UPS

This is a great exercise for your higher core muscles. It requires more movement than regular sit-ups and gets the heart pumping, which is always a bonus. Lie on your back and bring your knees and chest in towards each other at the same time, so your body is in a V shape. Make sure your feet don't touch the floor in between reps.

Beginner: 20 seconds non-stop and 40 seconds rest – 3–5 sets
Intermediate: 30 seconds non-stop and 30 seconds rest – 3–5 sets
Advanced: 40 seconds non-stop and 20 seconds rest – 3–5 sets

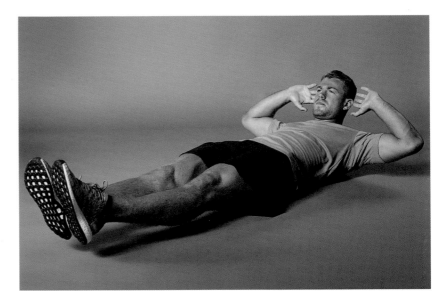

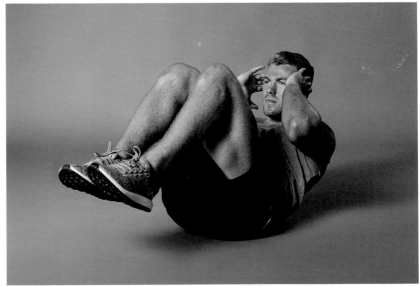

ELBOW TO KNEE CRUNCHES

Lie in a standard sit-up position but lift your feet off the ground. Now touch your elbow with the opposite knee as closely as possible. Do not let your feet touch the ground in between reps and make sure you really stretch to work the muscles.

Beginner: 20 seconds non-stop and 40 seconds rest – 3 5 sets
Intermediate: 30 seconds non-stop and 30 seconds rest – 3–5 sets
Advanced: 40 seconds non-stop and 20 seconds rest – 3–5 sets

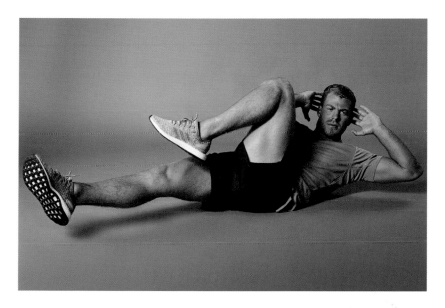

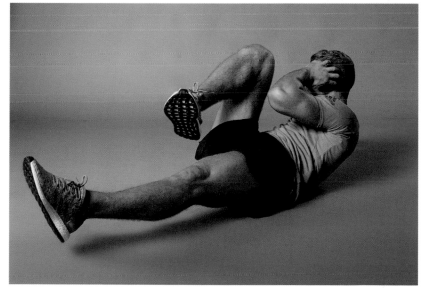

TRX EXERCISES

Can be done anywhere that has a stable structure to attach the equipment to.

TRX is similar to performing standard bodyweight exercises, but requires a lot more control, balance, strength, core strength and stability, since you're suspended off the ground while you do your workout. Essentially, it's the next level after standard bodyweight training, so it's best to give it a go once you've already made fitness a part of your routine, but you're looking for the next challenge. I often use this style of exercise on my footballer clients, as they require the ultimate core strength, stability and balance to prevent injury to other parts of the body. In particular, Theo Walcott saw vast improvements through this style of training.

My TRX trainer is one of the pieces of equipment that I always take away with me; it's super-light and easy to carry and can be fastened to any strong and stable structure, like a thick tree branch. These TRX exercises will take your core strength to the next level and improve your overall fitness.

PISTOL SQUATS

This exercise intensifies the standard squat position a little more. Make sure your feet are shoulder width apart, then squat down on one leg with the other leg straight in front, making sure you are holding on to the TRX.

Beginner: 10 reps on each leg, rest for 45 seconds – 3 sets
Intermediate: 12 reps on each leg, rest for 30 seconds – 3 sets
Advanced: 15 reps on each leg, rest for 30 seconds – 3 sets

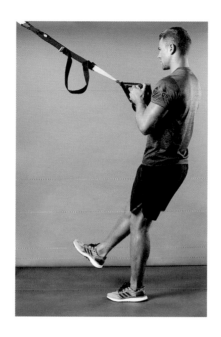
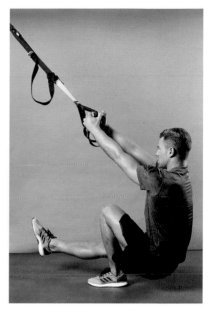

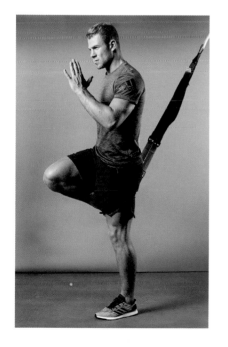
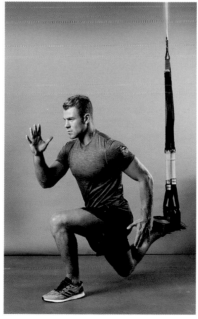

RUNNERS' LUNGES

Place one foot into the TRX loop – that is the foot you will be moving up and down in a right-angle position. Use the other leg to balance and control the move. When coming up from the lunge, make sure you bring the knee up to your chest, as if in a slow-motion running movement.

Beginner: 10 reps, rest for 45 seconds – 3 sets
Intermediate: 12 reps, rest for 30 seconds – 3 sets
Advanced: 15 reps, rest for 30 seconds – 3 sets

BICEP CURLS

Face the TRX, with your hands holding the loops firmly. Lean back slightly, bringing your feet forwards if necessary. Keep your elbows tight to your sides and bend in a right-angle motion, bringing your body backwards and forwards.

Beginner: 10 reps, rest for 45 seconds – 3 sets
Intermediate: 12 reps, rest for 30 seconds – 3 sets
Advanced: 15 reps, rest for 30 seconds – 3 sets

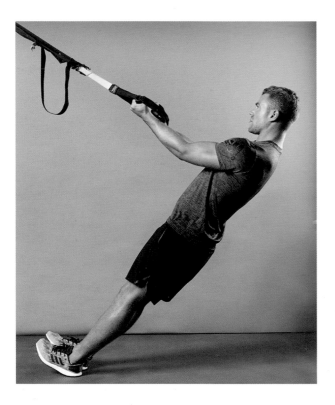
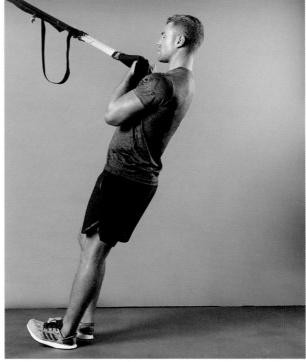

KNEE TUCKS

Use a fitness step to assist with this. Put both feet in the loops and stretch out your arms onto the fitness step so you are in a full plank position. Then bring both of your knees into your chest.

Beginner: 10 reps, rest for 45 seconds – 3 sets
Intermediate: 12 reps, rest for 30 seconds – 3 sets
Advanced: 15 reps, rest for 30 seconds – 3 sets

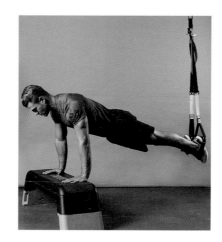
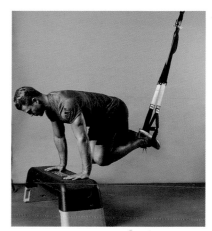

PIKES

Use a fitness step to assist with this. Put both feet in the loops and stretch your arms onto the fitness step so you are in a plank position. Engage your core and thrust your hips forwards, keeping your legs straight.

Beginner: 10 reps, rest for 45 seconds – 3 sets
Intermediate: 12 reps, rest for 30 seconds – 3 sets
Advanced: 15 reps, rest for 30 seconds – 3 sets

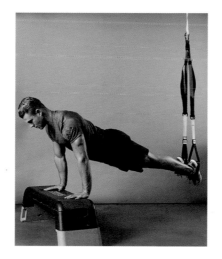
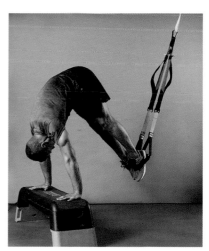

WEIGHT-TRAINING EXERCISES

Require equipment but very little space, ideal for toning and weight loss.

Weight-training exercise means using weights when exercising to encourage the muscles in your body to grow. Weight-training exercises are great for anyone whose goal is to tone up, gain lean muscle and create a more defined appearance. To do this style of exercise you'll have to buy some equipment or become familiar with the equipment in the gym. But you should never be afraid to ask a member of staff for assistance; the right technique is crucial to prevent injury and achieve the best results.

Please note: Weight training is suitable for both genders. Ladies, do not fear weights! Remember that by building muscle mass you are increasing your metabolic rate, which will help you burn more calories, even when chilling out. You will only ever BULK if you:

- Continuously increase the size of the weights you are using.

- Continuously increase the volume of reps or sets.

- Consume a lot of protein at the same time.

HOW DO I KNOW WHAT WEIGHT SIZE TO USE?

When using weights, you should be able to feel the burn in your muscles after completing sets in every single session. This means your routine is working. If it feels too easy you're not achieving anything. Get focused and push yourself!

I've separated the different weight exercises into the various muscle groups. You want to make sure you work on opposing muscle groups throughout the week so your body is in proportion and muscles get a chance to rest. I've also given you a suggested weight size, but bear in mind that everyone has different strengths so use this as a guideline.

WEIGHT EXERCISES FOR QUADS AND GLUTES

GOBLET SQUATS

Stand holding a light kettlebell by the horns close to your chest. This will be your starting position. Squat down with the kettlebell between your legs until your hamstrings are on your calves. Return to standing position and repeat.

Beginner: 10 reps, rest for 45 seconds – 3 sets (5kg)

Intermediate: 12 reps, rest for 30 seconds – 3 sets (7.5–10kg)

Advanced: 15 reps, rest for 30 seconds – 3 sets (10–20kg)

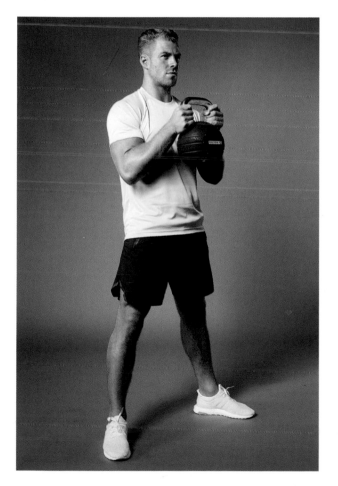

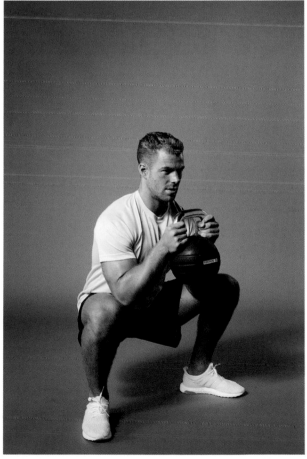

WEIGHTED BRIDGE

Lie on your back with your bum on the floor, then place a barbell on the pelvis area. Tighten your core and contract your glutes, then thrust your hips forwards and up, squeezing your glutes. Hold for a second, then slowly return to the floor.

Beginner: 10 reps, rest for 45 seconds – 3 sets (5kg)
Intermediate: 12 reps, rest for 30 seconds – 3 sets (7.5–10kg)
Advanced: 15 reps, rest for 30 seconds – 3 sets (10–20kg)

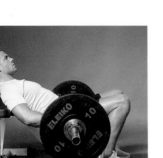

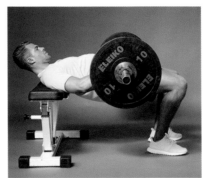

BARBELL REVERSE LUNGES

In a standing position, place a barbell across your shoulders, behind your head, holding it firmly with both hands. Slowly lunge, making sure your leg is at a right angle and you go down as low as possible. Do the same amount of reps on each leg, alternating the legs.

Beginner: 10 reps, rest for 45 seconds – 3 sets (5kg)
Intermediate: 12 reps, rest for 30 seconds – 3 sets (7.5–10kg)
Advanced: 15 reps, rest for 30 seconds – 3 sets (10–20kg)

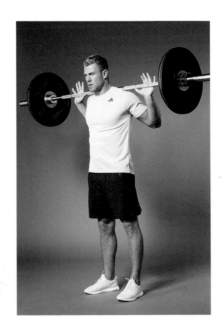

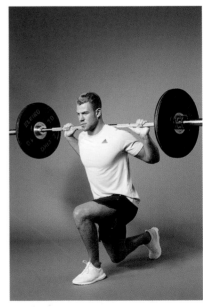

WEIGHT EXERCISES FOR HAMSTRINGS

STIFF LEG DEAD LIFT

Stand with your torso straight and your legs shoulder width apart, or slightly closer together if you prefer. Your knees should be slightly bent. Hold the barbell in front of you, hands shoulder width apart, with a strong grip (palms facing down). Keeping the knees stationary, lower the barbell to over the top of your feet by bending at the waist while keeping your back straight. Slowly and in a controlled manner, remembering to engage your core, rise back up to starting position, pause and repeat.

Beginner: 10 reps, rest for 45 seconds – 3 sets (10kg)
Intermediate: 12 reps, rest for 30 seconds – 3 sets (20kg)
Advanced: 15 reps, rest for 30 seconds – 3 sets (20kg+)

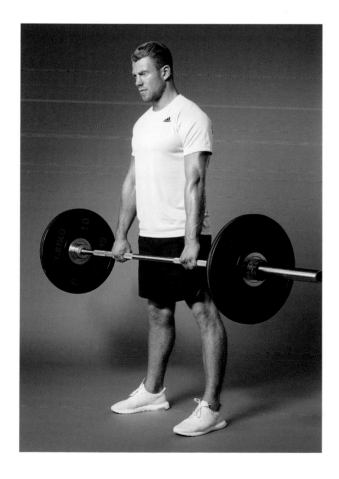

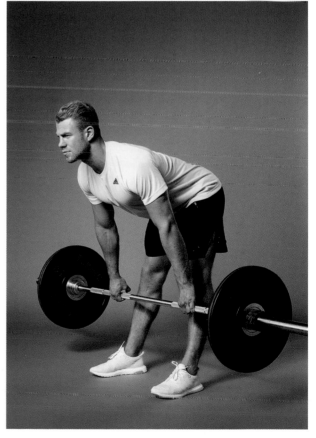

DUMBBELL SINGLE DEAD LIFT

Hold a dumbbell in each hand and position them down in front of your upper thighs with your arms straight. Stand with feet together, then lift one leg slightly so the foot is just off the floor. Then lean forwards keeping your back straight, lowering the dumbbells to the floor while also elevating your leg behind you so your torso and leg form a straight line. Slowly, whilst keeping your core and muscles engaged, return back to the starting position. Try and refrain from putting your lifted foot on the floor in order to enhance the exercise, giving you better results.

Beginner: 10 reps, rest for 45 seconds – 3 sets (5kg)

Intermediate: 12 reps, rest for 30 seconds – 3 sets (7.5–10kg)

Advanced: 15 reps, rest for 30 seconds – 3 sets (10–20kg)

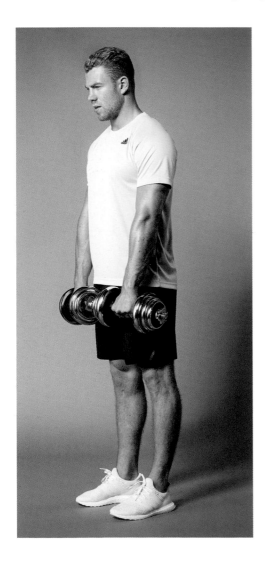
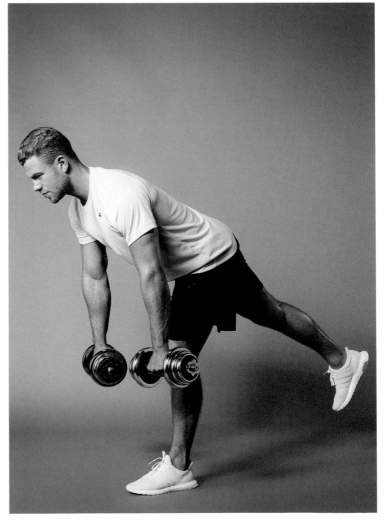

GOOD MORNINGS

Begin with a bar on a rack at shoulder height. Rack the bar across the rear of your shoulders as you would do for a power squat, not on top of your shoulders. Keep your back tight, shoulder blades pinched together and your knees slightly bent.

Begin by bending at the hips, moving them back as you bend over to near parallel position. Slowly, whilst keeping your core and muscles engaged, return back to the starting position with the weight in the same place.

Beginner: 10 reps, rest for 45 seconds – 3 sets (10kg)
Intermediate: 12 reps, rest for 30 seconds – 3 sets (20kg)
Advanced: 15 reps, rest for 30 seconds – 3 sets (20kg+)

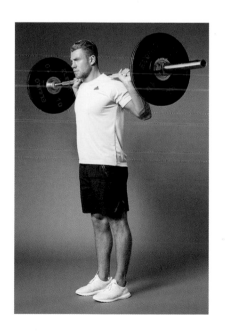
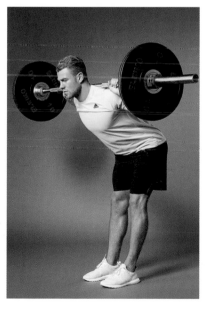
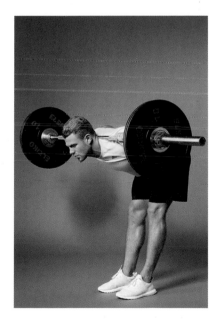

WEIGHT EXERCISES FOR THE BACK

BARBELL BENT-OVER ROW

Holding a barbell with hands shoulder-width apart and with a strong grip (palms facing down), bend your knees slightly and bring your torso forwards, by bending at the waist, while keeping the back straight until it is almost parallel to the floor. Now, while keeping the torso stationary, breathe out and lift the barbell towards you.

Beginner: 10 reps, rest for 45 seconds – 3 sets (10kg)
Intermediate: 12 reps, rest for 30 seconds – 3 sets (20kg)
Advanced: 15 reps, rest for 30 seconds – 3 sets (20kg+)

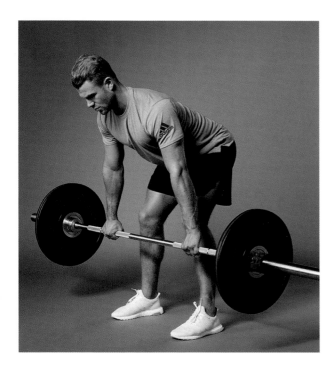
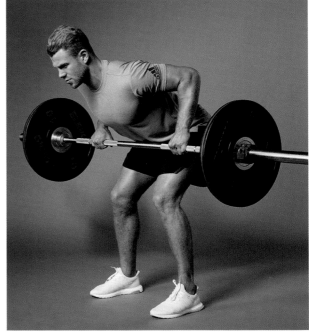

SINGLE ARM ROW

Choose a flat bench and place a dumbbell on either side of it. Kneel the right leg on top of the back of the bench with the other leg stabilising you standing on the floor, bend your torso forwards from the waist until your upper body is parallel to the floor, then place your right hand on the other end of the bench for support. Use the left arm to pull the dumbbell up to your armpit. Repeat on the other side.

Beginner: 10 reps, rest for 45 seconds – 3 sets per arm (10kg)
Intermediate: 12 reps, rest for 30 seconds – 3 sets per arm (20kg)
Advanced: 15 reps, rest for 30 seconds – 3 sets per arm (20kg+)

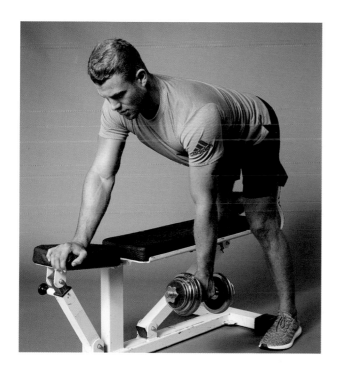
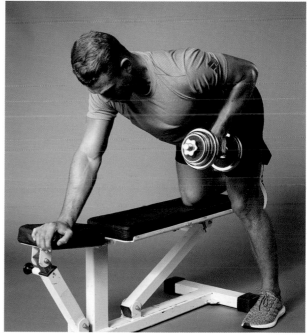

WEIGHT EXERCISES FOR BICEPS

BARBELL BICEP CURLS

Stand upright with your torso straight while holding a barbell at a shoulder-width grip, palms should be facing forwards. Whilst holding upper arms stationary and close to the body, curl the weights forwards, bending at the elbow.

Beginner: 10 reps, rest for 45 seconds – 3 sets (10kg)
Intermediate: 12 reps, rest for 30 seconds – 3 sets (20kg)
Advanced: 15 reps, rest for 30 seconds – 3 sets (20kg+)

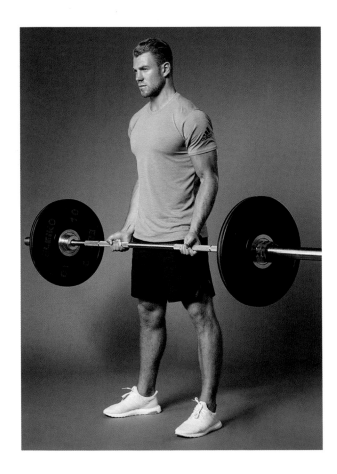 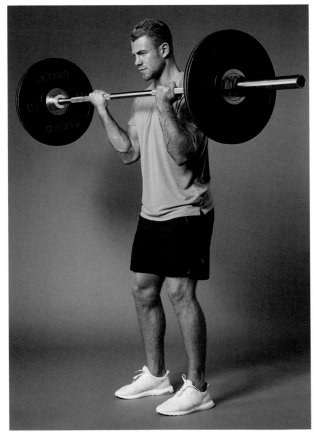

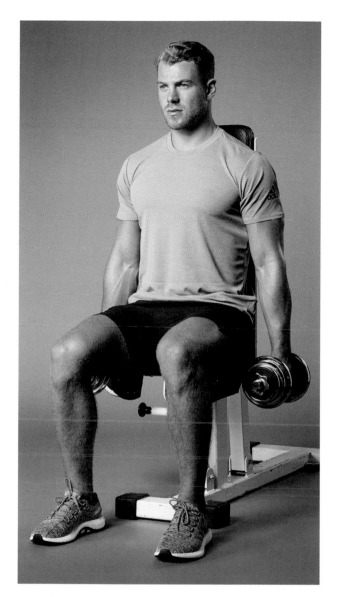
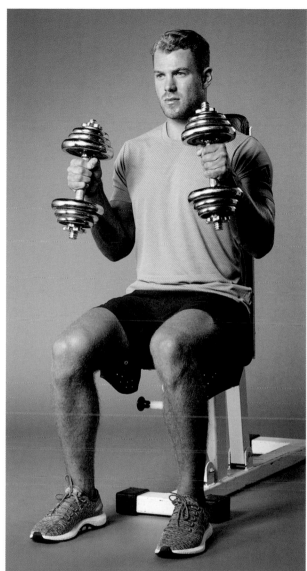

SEATED HAMMER CURLS

Sit down with a dumbbell in each hand, holding your upper arms stationary and close to the body, then curl the weights forwards, bending at the elbow.

Beginner: 10 reps, rest for 45 seconds – 3 sets (5kg per dumbbell)

Intermediate: 12 reps, rest for 30 seconds – 3 sets (10kg per dumbbell)

Advanced: 15 reps, rest for 30 seconds – 3 sets (20kg+ per dumbbell)

CONCENTRATION CURLS

Sit down on a flat bench with one dumbbell in front of you between your legs. Grab your dumbbell, palm facing up, then curl the weight forwards as you breathe out, resting the elbow of your arm on the inside of your thigh while holding the other arm stationary. Repeat with the other arm for an equal number of reps.

Beginner: 10 reps, rest for 45 seconds – 3 sets per arm (5kg per dumbbell)
Intermediate: 12 reps, rest for 30 seconds – 3 sets per arm (10kg per dumbbell)
Advanced: 15 reps, rest for 30 seconds – 3 sets per arm (20kg+ per dumbbell)

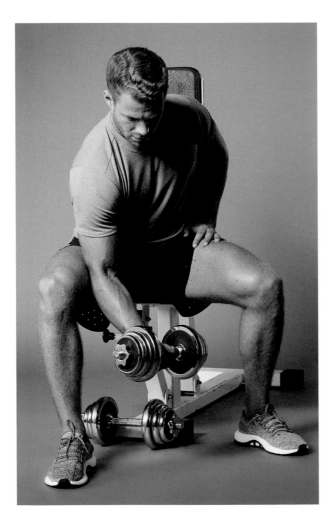

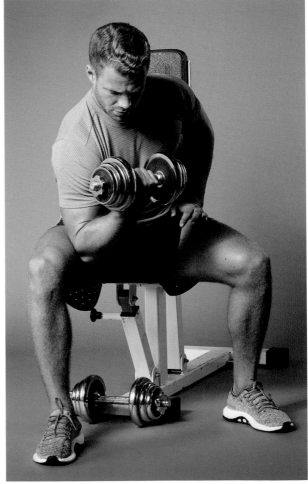

BARBELL BENCH PRESS

Lie back on a flat bench and, using a medium-width grip (a grip that creates a 90-degree angle in the middle of the movement between the forearms and the upper arms), lift the bar from the rack and hold up, holding it straight above you with your arms locked. Lower and repeat.

Beginner: 10 reps, rest for 45 seconds – 3 sets (20kg+)
Intermediate: 12 reps, rest for 30 seconds – 3 sets (30kg+)
Advanced: 15 reps, rest for 30 seconds – 3 sets (40kg+)

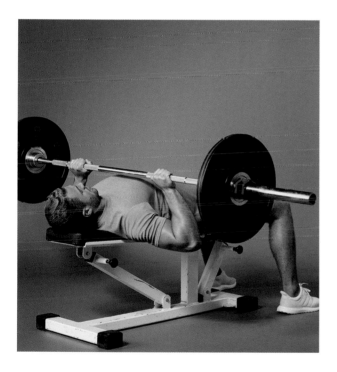
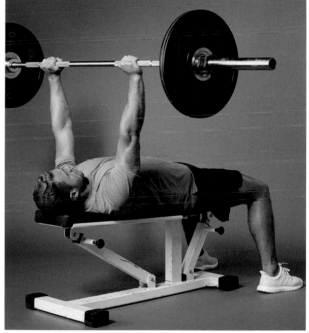

INCLINE DUMBBELL PRESS

Lie back on an incline bench with arms bent and out at your sides with a dumbbell in each hand, palms facing away from you. Then, in a slow, controlled movement, push the dumbbells up above you, shoulder width apart and level with the top of your chest.

Beginner: 10 reps, rest for 45 seconds – 3 sets (5kg per dumbbell)

Intermediate: 12 reps, rest for 30 seconds – 3 sets (10kg per dumbbell)

Advanced: 15 reps, rest for 30 seconds – 3 sets (20kg+ per dumbbell)

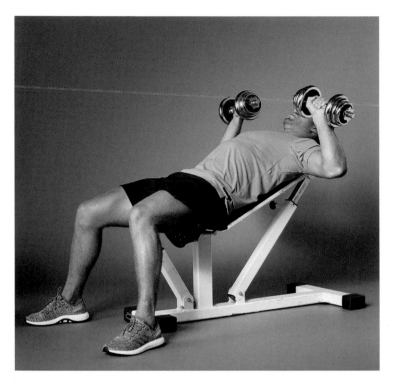

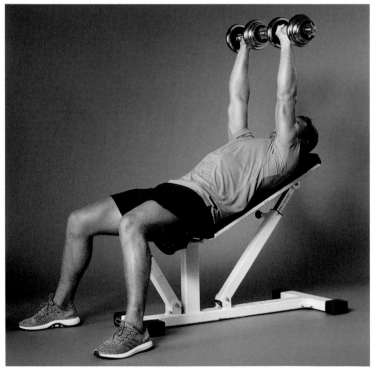

INCLINE DUMBBELL FLY

Hold a dumbbell in each hand and lie on an incline bench that is set to an angle of no more than 30 degrees. Extend your arms out at your sides with a slight bend at the elbows, hands facing your body, then bring your hands almost together above you, in a slow clapping motion, elbows still bent. Repeat.

Beginner: 10 reps, rest for 45 seconds – 3 sets (5kg per dumbbell)

Intermediate: 12 reps, rest for 30 seconds – 3 sets (10kg per dumbbell)

Advanced: 15 reps, rest for 30 seconds – 3 sets (20kg+ per dumbbell)

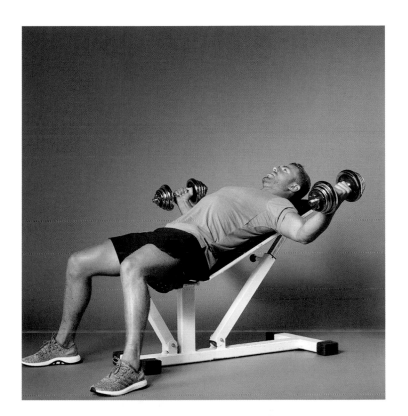

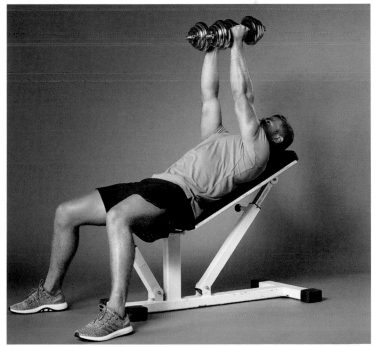

WEIGHT EXERCISES FOR SHOULDERS

SEATED SHOULDER PRESS

Sit comfortably on a press bench or utility bench with a dumbbell in each hand. Propel the dumbbells into position, palms facing forward and elbows at a right angle on either side of you. This is your starting position. Push the dumbbells straight up and then slowly and controlled, bring the dumbbells down to starting position. Repeat.

Beginner: 10 reps, rest for 45 seconds – 3 sets (5kg per dumbbell)

Intermediate: 12 reps, rest for 30 seconds – 3 sets (10kg per dumbbell)

Advanced: 15 reps, rest for 30 seconds – 3 sets (20kg+ per dumbbell)

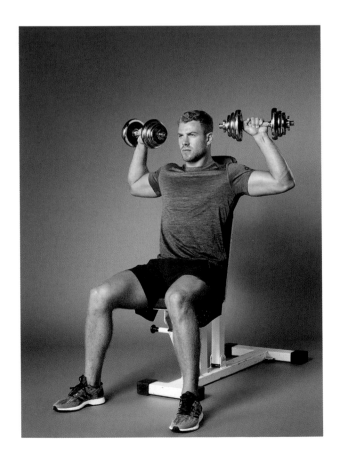

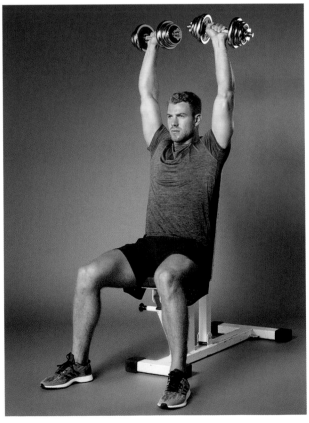

LATERAL RAISE

In a standing position with your feet firmly placed for balance, grasp a dumbbell in each hand. Hold the dumbbells hanging straight down at your sides, your palms facing down and your elbows slightly bent. Raise both dumbbells simultaneously directly up by the sides of your body until they are level with your armpit, then lower and repeat.

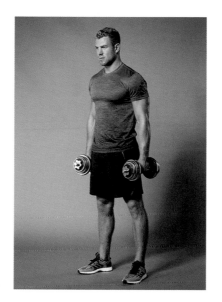

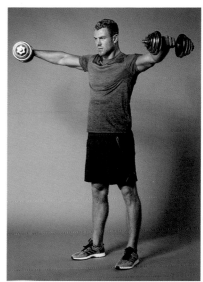

Beginners: 10 reps, rest for 45 seconds – 3 sets (5kg per dumbbell)

Intermediate: 12 reps, rest for 30 seconds – 3 sets (10kg per dumbbell)

Advanced: 15 reps, rest for 30 seconds – 3 sets (20kg+ per dumbbell)

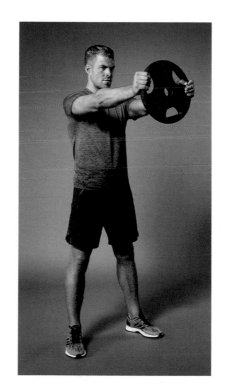

PLATE FRONTAL RAISE

Hold a weight plate directly in front of you, making sure your arms are completely straight, your feet are shoulder-width apart and your back is straight. Hold this position for the recommended time.

Beginners: 30 seconds non-stop and 45 seconds rest – 3 sets (5kg+)

Intermediate: 45 seconds non-stop and 30 seconds rest – 3 sets (10kg+)

Advanced: 60 seconds non-stop and 30 seconds rest – 3 sets (15kg+)

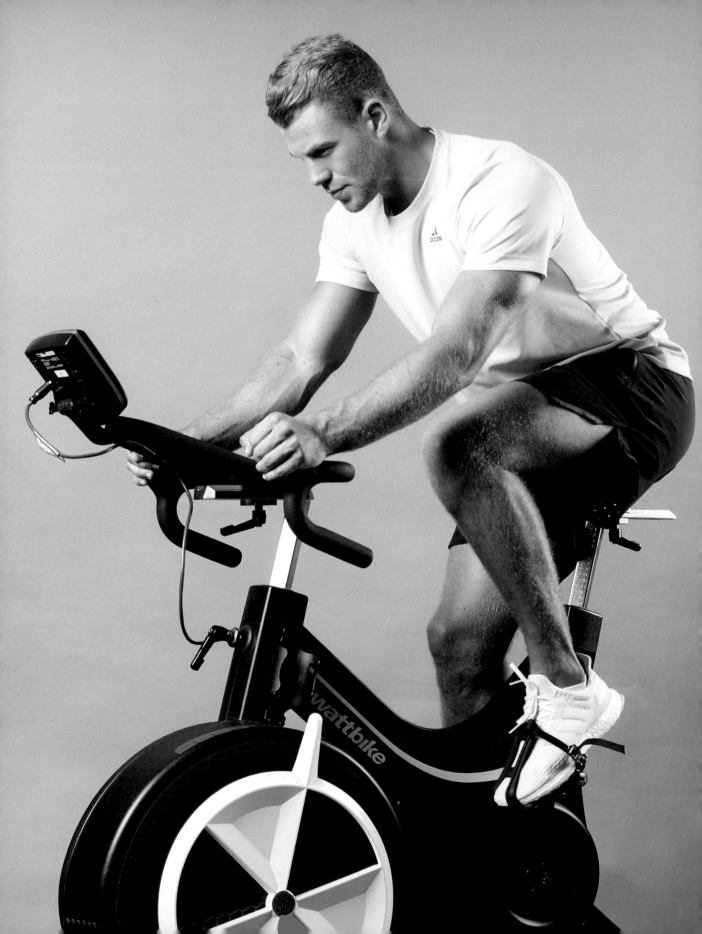

CIRCUIT TRAINING

Ideal for indoors or outdoors but requires a medium-size space and preferably equipment.

Circuit training, in my opinion, is one of the most effective and enjoyable ways to get in a full body workout incorporating both bodyweight and weight-training exercises. It's basically several stations with different exercises at each that you rotate round, usually with one or more fitness buddies. Circuits are my signature exercise style, and I use them with Toni Terry, Louise Redknapp and my sister Connie and they've all seen incredible results. In groups you can spur each other on, get into teams and compete against each other. It's fast-paced so time flies by and there's lots of variety so you don't get bored.

Try building your own circuit using the exercises on the previous pages. Ten stations including exercises targeting muscle groups in your upper body, your core and your legs is usually a good shout. You can either do all bodyweight exercises or incorporate some weight-training exercises in there if you like. Each person starts at a station and works their way round, completing it twice or three times depending on their fitness levels and the time available.

ROUND 1	ROUND 2
45 seconds on	30 seconds on
30 seconds rest	10 seconds rest
Move to the next station	Move to the next station
Repeat on every station	Repeat on every station
Rest for 2 minutes after whole circuit completion	Rest for 2 minutes and repeat once more

HIIT

Can be completed anywhere, but I prefer using a treadmill.

High-intensity interval training (HIIT) has exploded in popularity in the last couple of years, and for all the right reasons. All it means is giving 100 percent in a short space of time (30–45 seconds) with small rest periods in between (10–30 seconds). It's the quickest way to burn fat.

HIIT WORKOUT BEGINNER	HIIT WORKOUT INTERMEDIATE	HIIT WORKOUT ADVANCED
5-minute incline fast walk at speed 6km/h	5-minute jog on speed 12km/h	5-minute jog on speed 15km/h
5-minute jog on speed 10km/h	Rest for 1 minute	Walk for 60 seconds at 6km/h
Rest for 1 minute	Increase speed to 14km/h	Increase speed to 18km/h
Increase speed to 12km/h	Run for 60 seconds on, 60 seconds off x 4	Run for 60 seconds on, 60 seconds off x 4
Run for 60 seconds on, 60 seconds off x 5	Increase speed to 16km/h	Increase speed to 20–22km/h
	Run for 30 seconds on, 30 seconds off x 5	Run for 30 seconds on, 30 seconds off x 5
	Walk for 2 minutes at speed 4km/h	Walk for 2 minutes at speed 4km/h

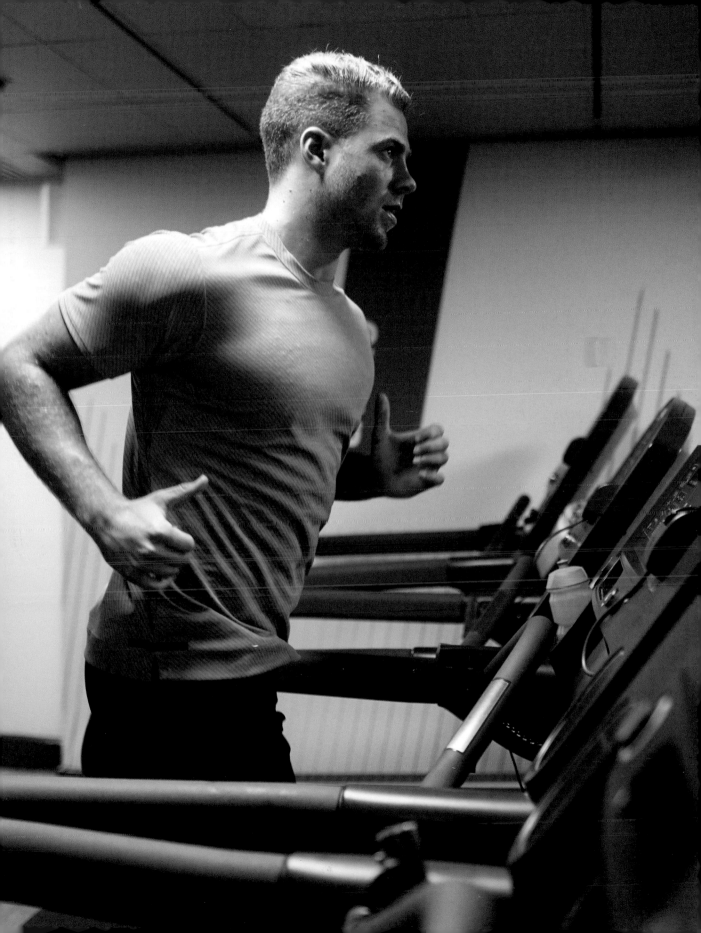

OTHER EXERCISES TO ENJOY

BOXING

Boxing requires the right technique to prevent injury but once you've nailed that, you're sorted. Either find a personal trainer specialising in boxing or search for local boxercise, boxing or kick-boxing classes in your area. I love boxing and always try to incorporate it into sessions with clients – as long as they enjoy it. Boxing using gloves and pads has so many awesome benefits. It's a great way to burn fat, improve fitness levels, build muscle and it can also help you to de-stress – there's nothing more satisfying than punching the pads on a bad day!

There's something truly satisfying about feeling strong and fierce. You also work loads of muscle groups as you twist, reach and constantly move around on your toes and you can burn around 600 calories in 45 minutes of intense boxing. It's ideal for anyone who's competitive or enjoys fast-paced workouts and sports.

GYM CLASSES

If exercising at home or in the park doesn't work for you, seriously consider joining a gym that offers classes at no extra cost. That way, you're less likely to leave mid-workout, you're motivated by the instructor and you have the opportunity to meet like-minded people. Try spinning, yoga, body pump, boxercise, Pilates, circuits or Legs, Bums and Tums – there's something for everyone and for every goal.

WEIGHT-LOSS CLASSES

If losing weight is your primary goal, high-intensity cardio-based classes such as spinning, circuits, dance and swimming/water aerobics are your best bet. Never be afraid to tell the instructor before the class starts that you're new; that way they're aware of your fitness levels and can give you some extra support during the session. If the instructor isn't as tough as me you'll need to push yourself! Remember, only you can know when you're really giving it everything you have.

TONING AND MUSCLE GAIN

Classes such as body pump, boxercise and TRX are great for this as you'll also learn so many new techniques that you can use in your own gym sessions.

Remember, even though you're looking to gain muscle, you still want to be sweating and increasing your heart rate in these sessions, so choose classes that are more weight- or strength-orientated with bursts of cardio.

FLEXIBILITY, RELAXATION AND MENTALITY

If one of your goals is to de-stress, relax more or improve flexibility and stability through exercise, classes such as yoga and Pilates are brilliant. Many football clubs incorporate yoga or Pilates sessions to help stretch and improve core strength. These sorts of exercises are low intensity and focus more on strength and toning. They also encourage you to meditate – the perfect type of exercise for rest days and stressful times.

STRETCHING AND RECOVERY

Rest days are essential – you must give your body time to repair to prevent injury from the hard work you've put in.

STRETCHING

Warming up the body BEFORE a session is essential to loosen and prepare your muscles ready for a workout. Don't stretch cold – always start with some gentle movement such as jogging on the spot. It's also important to stretch AFTER a session as muscles can become tight and fatigued. Stretching after every session will, over time, elongate your muscles and help you appear more slender. Stretching after weight training in particular is extremely important as this style of exercise puts most strain on our muscles. There are a variety of simple stretches you should complete before and after every session.

CALVES

Get onto all fours, lean back onto your toes, wrap one foot around the other (just below the calf muscle) and lean back further onto your toes. You should feel the stretch in the calf. Swap legs and repeat.

QUADS

Lie down on your side, resting on your elbow, body straight and elongated. Bend the top leg backwards and hold with the matching arm and hold. Swap sides and repeat until your quads feel looser.

HIP FLEXOR

Kneel down with your body upright. Place one knee in front forming a right angle, so one leg is in front of the other kneeling. Or place your hands on your hips and slowly push forwards and return back to the original position.

GROIN STRETCH

Sit down on the floor and place your feet together with knees in the air forming a diamond shape. Hold your ankles and gently press the knees down with your elbows to stretch the groin.

LOWER BACK

1 Lie on your tummy with your feet flat. Lift your upper body upwards so your hands are flat on the ground and your arms are straight. Gently push to feel the stretch. Your chin should be facing forwards, looking ahead.

2 Lie on your back, bend your knees into your chest and turn your bent legs right or left so they are flat on the floor, ensuring your back is still flat and your arms are spread out to help keep your back flat.

UPPER BACK

Get onto all fours with your hands under your shoulders and your knees under your hips. Keeping your hands and knees cemented into the ground, arch your back, hold for 10 seconds, relax and repeat.

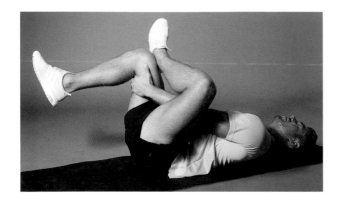

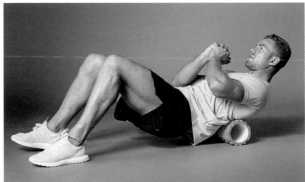

GLUTES

Lie on your back, bring one knee into your chest and hold with your hands. Bend the other leg and place on top. Gently pull the bent leg towards you. Swap legs.

UPPER BODY

1 Put one arm across your chest and hook it with the opposite arm. Using the hooking arm push the horizontal arm more closely to your chest to feel the stretch.

2 Raise one arm above your head and then bend at the elbow so your arm is bent behind the head. With the other arm push down the elbow with your opposite hand.

FOAM ROLLER

Foam rolling or self-myofascial release is a form of stretching. It focuses on the pressure points in the body and helps to release tightness allowing your muscles to return back to normal performance.

With a foam roller the aim is to place pressure on the muscle – whether that is your calf, glutes, quads, back or arms – and roll backwards and forwards on the foam roller. This will stretch out the muscle – the tighter the muscle the more painful it can be but you may have to grit your teeth and bear it – stretching your muscles is essential for your performance and to prevent injury.

PROTEIN

Don't forget to tuck into a good source of lean protein after your workout – either a good-quality protein powder or a delicious meal. As your body is still burning calories after your session, you also need a small amount of carbs to refuel and work alongside the protein. You get the very best results and your body is prepped for the next session.

LOVE AND DEDICATION BUT NOT OBSESSION

If you are finding ways to exercise and work out seven days a week, slow down. You need at least one day to relax your muscles and enjoy other things. On the other hand, if exercise isn't your thing at the moment but you're finding the motivation to start, then that's amazing.

Wherever you are on your journey, don't get obsessed, don't feel guilty for having a day off and definitely don't sacrifice everything else in your life to simply squeeze in exercise.

Yes, exercise needs to become a priority, but always be mindful of your limits and abilities, and remember to ENJOY IT.

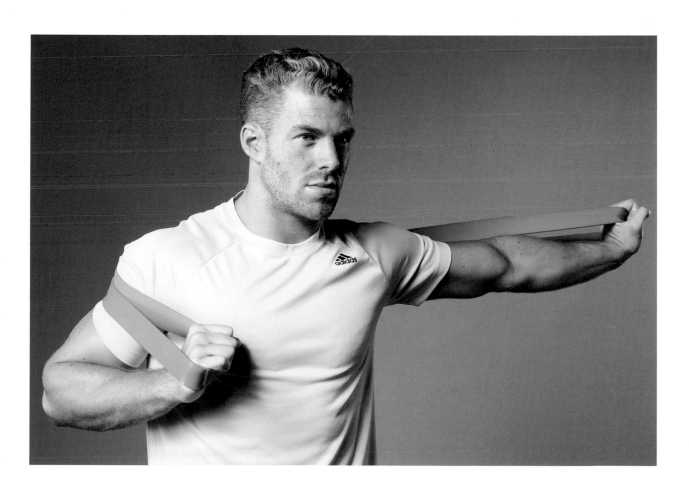

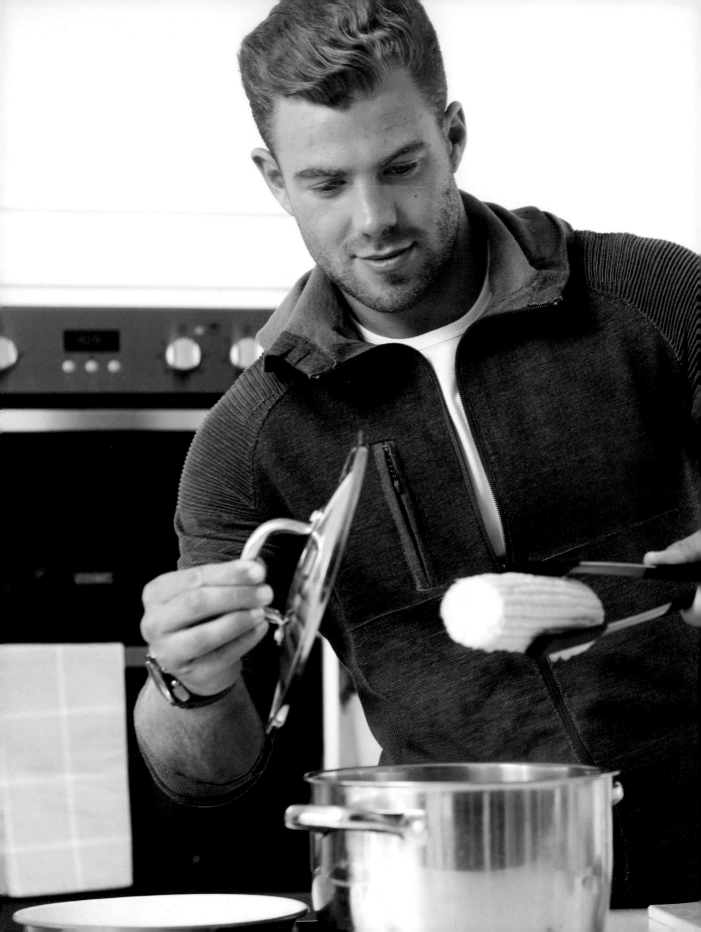

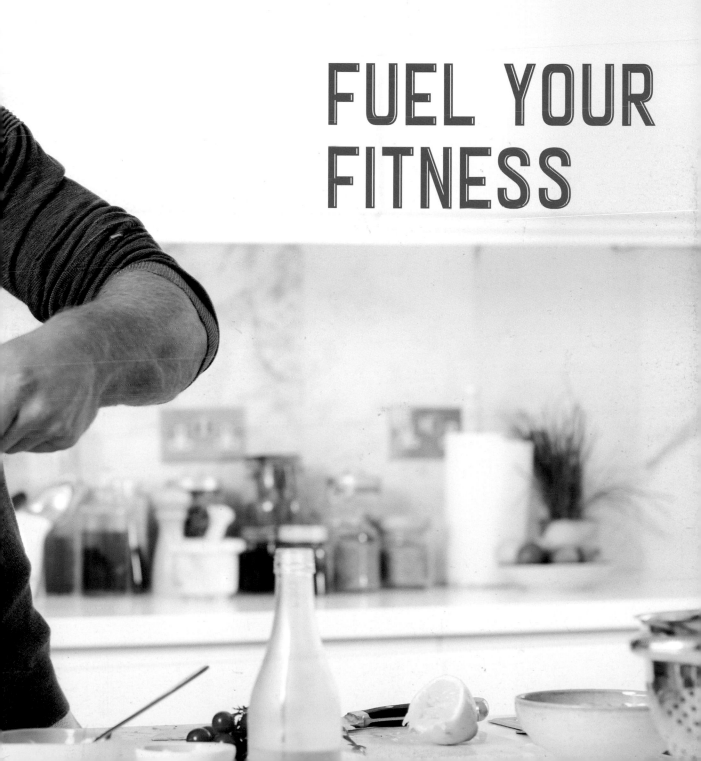

CHAPTER 3

FUEL YOUR FITNESS

'You wouldn't fill an unleaded car with diesel, so why fill your body with the wrong fuel?'

That comparison might sound a bit extreme, but it makes my point. Our bodies don't know how to properly break down unnatural, processed food and drink, which is why it leaves us feeling run-down and sluggish.

What we eat and drink also has a huge impact on the energy and motivation we need to lead a more active lifestyle. To feel good, it's vital that the majority of the time (90 per cent) you eat nutrient-dense, colourful meals that contain the right balance of fats, proteins, complex carbs and plants.

GIVE YOURSELF THE GIFT OF ENERGY

If you rarely have the energy to exercise, eating the right food could change everything. Ingredients that release energy slowly into the bloodstream keep us feeling fuller for longer and more energised and usually contain lots of healthy fibre. This is why no-carb diets can be quite exhausting! Take an honest look at how much sugar and caffeine you're taking in – it could offer a clue to your yo-yoing energy. Another reason might be that you're not getting enough sleep. If you've taken steps to address all of these things and you're still not feeling any perkier, I'd recommend consulting a nutritionist. Having the energy to keep fit is the first and most crucial step.

Once you've overcome the first hurdle and have got out there to exercise, you'll find that being active can help to give you that burst of energy you've been missing. Lethargy or lacking energy can become a vicious cycle: we lose motivation so we skip the gym and instead go home and eat a convenient dinner, slob around, go to bed. Then the next day we go to work, sit at a desk, snack all day, feel lethargic, skip the gym again… It's up to you to break the cycle; you need to dig deep and push yourself – and your diet is the place to start.

BACK TO THE WORD BALANCE

Getting the right balance in your lifestyle is key to feeling good. For some people, one wholesome meal becomes such an achievement that they think they can then reward themselves for the rest of the day with unhealthy treats. We need to take our eating habits far more seriously. How do you do this? Here are some of my top tips:

- Make food from scratch and add flavour using spices and herbs. Don't reach for the over-sugared, processed sauces in a jar.

- Be more creative in the kitchen and get kitted out with some healthy cookbooks to inspire your meals.

- Get your children involved in shopping for food and cooking it. Education is key for healthy eating – and you can't start too early.

- Plan ahead when it comes to the weekly food shop; decide what recipe you want to cook, write a shopping list and stick to it, then you won't be grabbing convenience foods in a supermarket dash.

- Learn to enjoy foods that nourish your body – having the right mindset is everything.

It's up to us to take responsibility for looking beyond the convenience foods in the supermarket – even more so if you're the one who does the food shop for the whole family. The choices you make don't just affect you but your family too. Balance is also about how much you eat. Quantities should be flexed up or down depending on how and when you're exercising, as well as how much you move around day to day.

SO IF I EXERCISE I CAN EAT WHAT I WANT?

Don't become the 'I've exercised so I can eat what I want,' person, though. Your metabolism doesn't work at the speed of light and metabolic rates vary from person to person, so be mindful of this or seek advice from a qualified nutritionist if you want to know more about your own personal metabolic rate.

Many people believe that exercising gives them an excuse to indulge later and they consider this approach to be a healthy balance. As long as they exercise 3–5 times a week, they can eat and drink whatever they want, and perhaps use the time after a gym session to indulge in a cheat meal or sugary snack.

I'm not a fan of this approach. Yes, exercise helps you burn fat, improves your fitness levels and makes you feel good about yourself, but it doesn't give you all the vitamins, minerals, essential fatty acids, protein and fibre that you get from the right food. If you want to treat yourself, use the post workout period to whip up a slap-up meal with lean protein and complex carbohydrates, like sweet potato and brown rice.

If you're reading this and you haven't noticed changes in your body or health despite doing more exercise, you might want to look at your what you're eating.

IF I EAT AFTER EXERCISING, IS IT A WASTE OF TIME?

While some people make the mistake of eating too much of the wrong food, others don't eat enough food in general. Don't get stuck in the mindset that if you eat after you've exercised you'll be taking back all the calories you've just worked off. This is categorically not true.

Your body not only burns calories during an exercise session, it also burns them after a workout, during its recovery period. Whatever you eat post-workout contributes to the repair and re-growth of muscles and gives you back your energy so you can get on with your day. It's essential, and it doesn't make you put on weight, so long as you eat the right food in the right quantities.

So getting the right balance is key, and only you can make that happen. Reminding yourself of the goal you set in the previous chapters should keep you motivated and on track with eating well. Exercise and the right food work hand in hand, and if you want to achieve the best, most sustainable results you need both, which leads me on perfectly to my favourite recipes!

MY RECIPES

My style of cooking is super-simple and a dish rarely takes longer than 30 minutes to prepare, cook and devour. I'm super-busy and always on the go, like most people, so while I do discourage eating convenience food, I'm also realistic about the demands of modern life. I appreciate that most meals need to be time- and cost-effective – as well as healthy. I've seen the results, too, and I know it is the key to sustaining a healthy lifestyle in the long term.

My recipes are inspired by exactly what I like to eat at home – by myself or with friends and family – but I've also included a few extra indulgences for the weekends. Although I have a no-nonsense approach to healthy eating and exercise, I do appreciate how tough it is to resist all the temptation around us, so hopefully my social sharers, sweet treats and sugar-free cocktails will help curb any sugar cravings!

THE ESSENTIALS

Here are my top tips to take on board before you start this new way of eating:

- Clear out your cupboards and fridge of anything processed and sugary. If you don't like waste, take it to your local food bank. You have to start not only with a clear mind but also a clear kitchen.

- Be ready to retrain your taste buds – you're about to pack in some serious vitamins and minerals!

- Invest in a good spice rack – I use lots of spices to add flavour and keep food exciting yet still nutrient-dense. Remember, ready-made jarred sauces are usually packed with sugar, salt and preservatives, so making your own keeps you in control of what's going into your body.

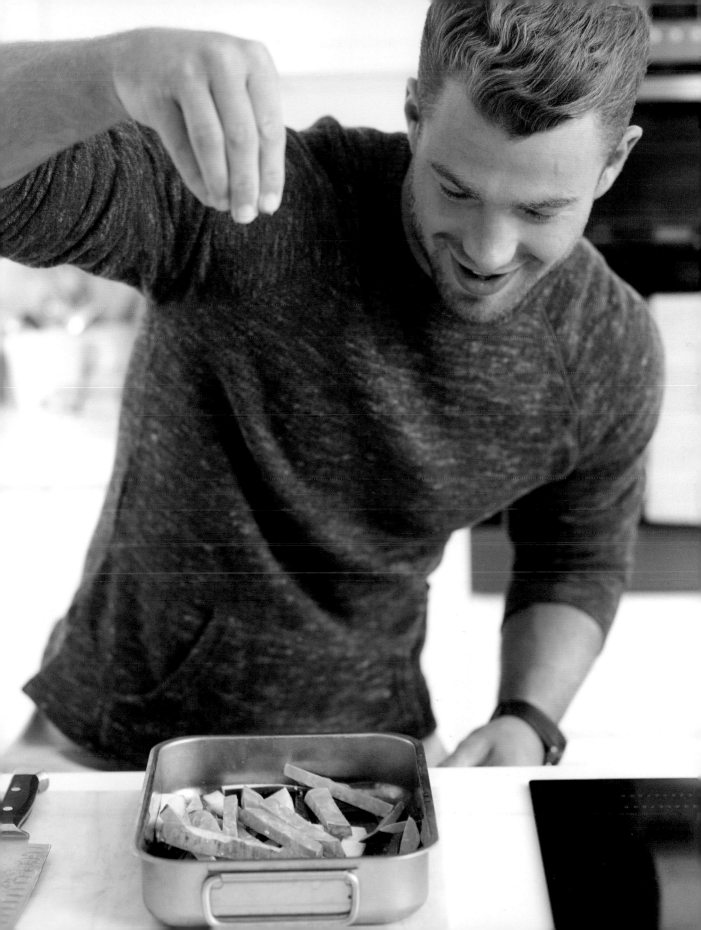

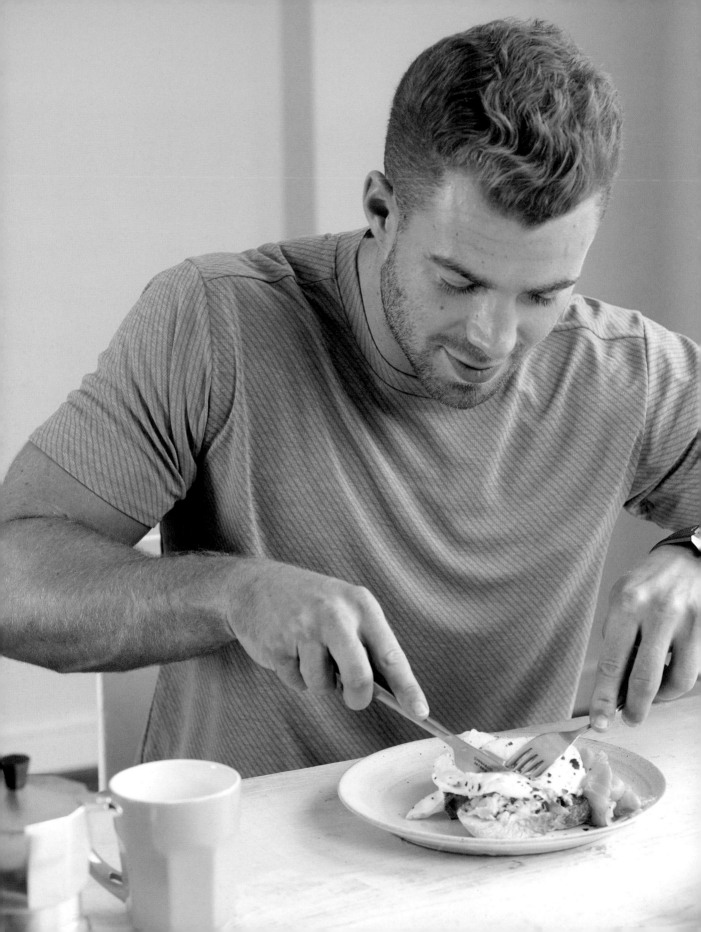

BREAKFAST

Eat breakfast like a king,
lunch like a prince and
dinner like a pauper.

Start each day with a good breakfast to kick start
your metabolism – no exceptions. What you eat
in the morning can determine your mood, insulin
levels and appetite for the rest of the day. So make
sure you're eating slow-releasing carbs, good fats,
protein and fibre, which will keep you full and
energised.

THREE-EGG OMELETTE WITH SPINACH, TOMATOES AND A SPRINKLE OF FETA

This is a great protein-rich breakfast, packed with essential fats and greens. You can make any sort of omelette with the leftover veggies in your fridge, so use whatever you have – just keep it colourful.

3 medium eggs
1 tsp coconut oil
8 cherry tomatoes, halved
handful of baby spinach leaves
20g feta cheese, crumbled
sea salt and freshly ground black
    pepper

1   Whisk the eggs in a bowl until well combined and season with a pinch of salt and pepper.

2   Heat the oil in a non-stick frying pan over a medium-high heat and add the cherry tomatoes (or any other chopped veg you have) .

3   Once the tomatoes have softened and gone a little brown, after about 3 minutes, add the spinach, and leave to wilt. This will only take about a minute. Remove the veg from the pan, reduce the heat to medium-low and pour in the eggs, moving them around the pan for an even finish.

4   Let the eggs gently cook for 2–3 minutes.

5   Sprinkle on the spinach, tomatoes and feta and let them sink into the remaining raw egg.

6   Gently fold the omelette in half whilst in the pan so the heat can travel through, then shake the omelette onto your plate and enjoy.

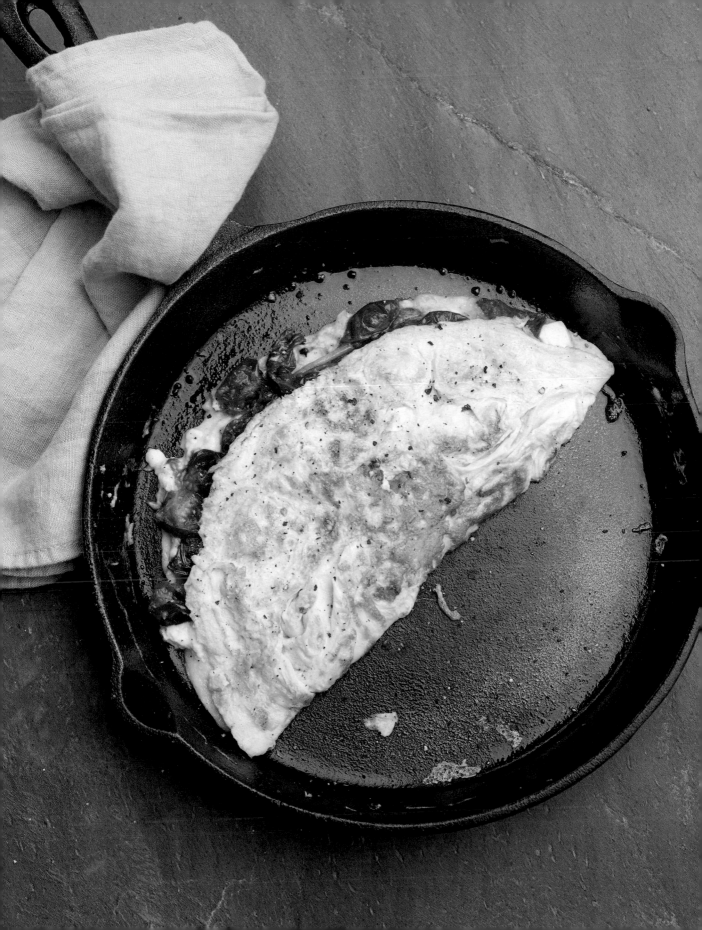

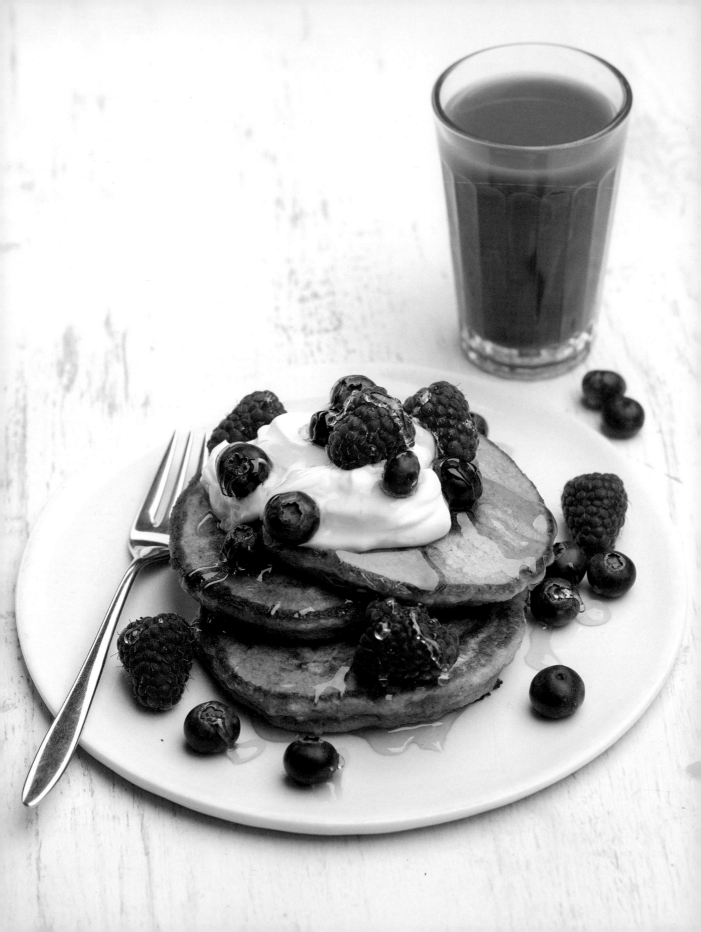

ONE-CUP PROTEIN PANCAKES WITH PICK 'N' MIX TOPPINGS

If you like pancakes, you'll love these. They make a great breakfast or brunch for the weekend or you can prepare them the night before and heat them up in the toaster the following morning. Add your favourite toppings and you'll be in heaven.

FOR THE BATTER
80g rolled oats
1 medium egg
¼ tsp baking powder
1 tsp vanilla extract
1 banana
2 tsp coconut oil

FOR THE TOPPINGS (CHOOSE UP TO 3)
fresh berries
10g dark chocolate chips
1 tbsp whipped Greek yoghurt
1 tbsp honey
handful of crushed nuts

1   Add the oats to a blender and blitz to a flour texture, then add all the other batter ingredients except the coconut oil and blitz under smooth and creamy.

2   Add the coconut oil to a non-stick frying pan and pour a third of the mixture into the pan. Cook over a medium heat on each side for 3–4 minutes until brown but not burnt. Repeat to make three pancakes, each about 8cm wide.

3   Stack your pancakes, load on your chosen toppings and enjoy!

RUNNY EGG WITH GREEN AND BROWN SOLDIERS

Eggs and soldiers was a classic breakfast growing up. I loved it, too, so I just had to make my own adult version.

2 large eggs
4 asparagus spears
1 slice of sourdough bread
2 slices of Parma ham (optional)
1 tsp butter

1 Add the eggs to a pan of water and bring the water up to the boil – for the perfect runny yolk I set the timer for 3 minutes at the point of it bubbling. Boil the asparagus in the same pan for 5 minutes to save on washing up.

2 Add the sourdough to the toaster.

3 Remove the eggs and put into egg cups, removing the tops to prevent over-cooking, then remove the asparagus spears.

4 Wrap the Parma ham around two of the cooked asparagus. Butter the toasted sourdough, then slice into 1cm thick strips and plate up next to the asparagus.

5 Now dip your green and brown soldiers into the eggs, and don't forget to eat the egg whites once the yolks are all gone!

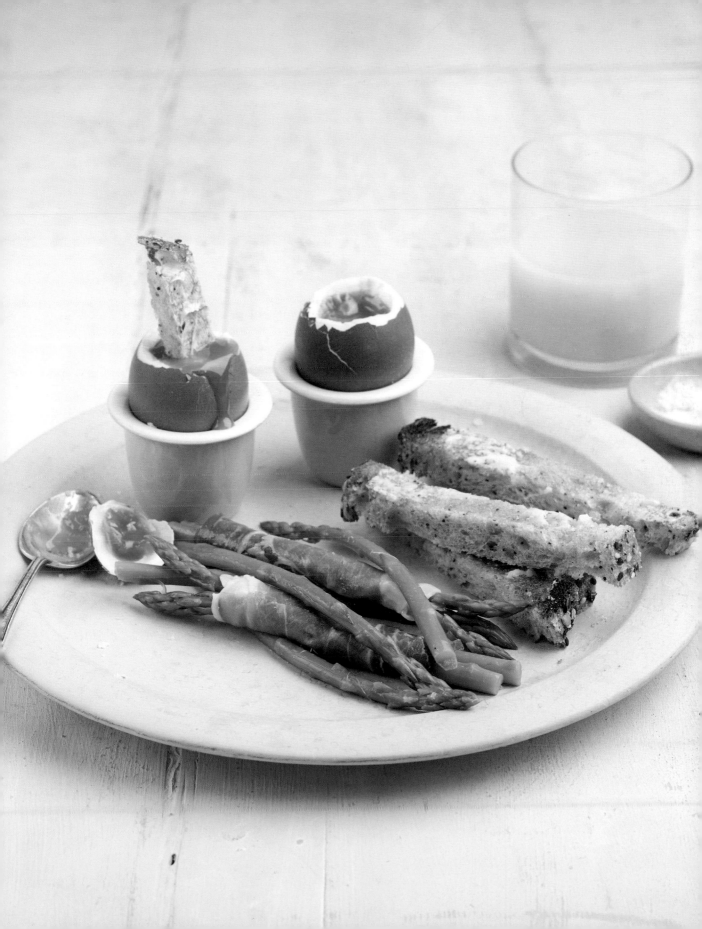

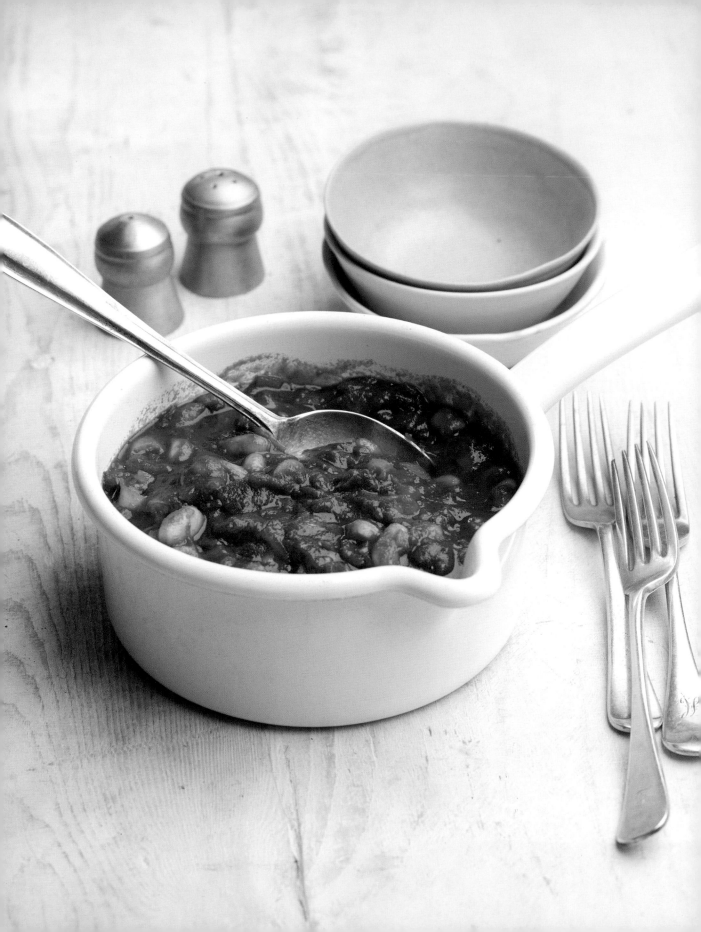

BRAD'S BAKED BEAN PROTEIN POT

This breakfast is a hug in a bowl – super comforting and delicious yet nutritious. The beans can be made the night before, then served in a bowl or spooned over toast – you'll have enough for 4 servings

FOR THE BEANS

1 onion, peeled and diced
1 tbsp olive oil
1 garlic clove, peeled and crushed
1 x 400g tin of cannellini or mixed
    beans, drained and rinsed
2 x 400g tins of chopped tomatoes
1 tsp paprika
splash of Worcestershire sauce or
    balsamic vinegar
pinch of sea salt and freshly ground
    black pepper

FOR THE REST OF THE POT

2 slices of good-quality bacon,
    trimmed
1 large egg
1 tsp coconut oil

1   Sweat the onion in a medium saucepan with the olive oil over a medium-low heat for 8–10 minutes until soft, then add the crushed garlic and stir.

2   Add the beans and stir, then add the tinned tomatoes, stir and let simmer over a medium heat for 30 minutes.

3   During the last 5 minutes of the beans simmering and thickening, dry-fry your trimmed bacon until crisp, then fry the egg in the coconut oil.

4   Return to your beans for seasoning, add the paprika, Worcestershire sauce or balsamic vinegar and salt and pepper and stir for another 2–3 minutes.

5   Either plate up a quarter of the beans, the bacon and egg over a slice of wholemeal toast or layer the bacon, egg and a quarter of the beans in a bowl or Tupperware for a flavoursome and filling breakfast on the go.

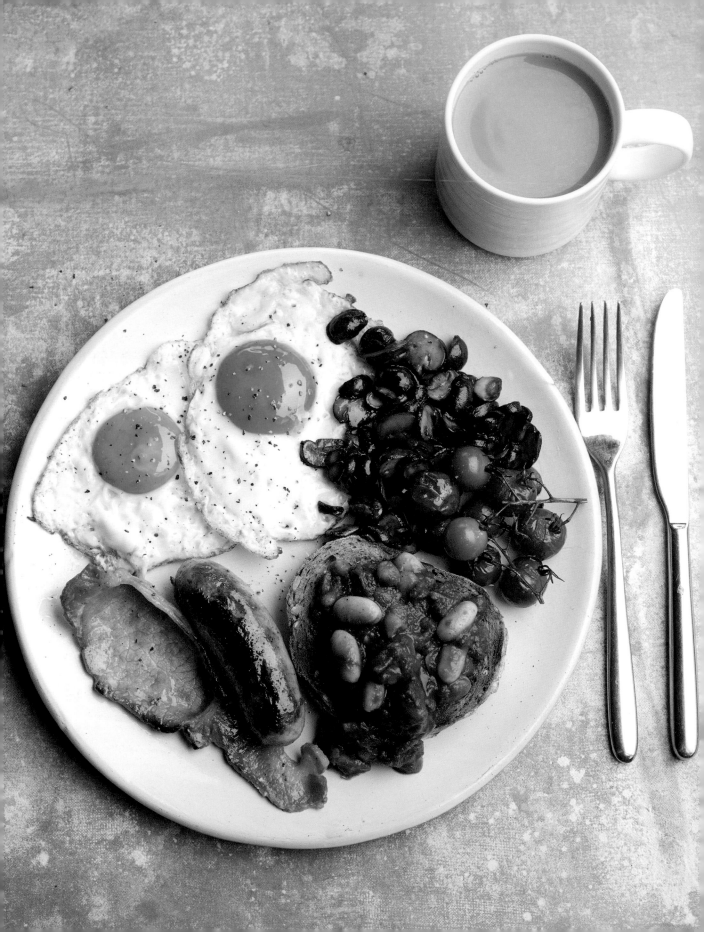

FIT FULL ENGLISH

I had to include the traditional full English since it's practically a national treasure, but I've added my own twist to this classic, making it the perfect balanced breakfast for weekends and for the whole family.

2 tsp coconut oil
1 good-quality turkey or pork sausage (97% pork)
1 slice of good-quality bacon, trimmed
6 chestnut mushrooms
6 cherry tomatoes
2 spoonfuls of my homemade baked beans (see page 121 and prepare a little in advance)
2 eggs
1 slice of wholemeal or seeded bread

NOTE
If you are vegetarian you can swap the sausage for a veggie sausage and add avocado and spinach to your plate instead of bacon.

1   Put 1 teaspoon of the coconut oil into a non-stick frying pan, add the sausage and fry over a medium-high heat until brown all over, then add the bacon. Leave them over a medium-low heat for 20–25 minutes, or until the sausage is completely cooked through and the bacon is crisp, turning often. In the meantime prepare the other ingredients.

2   Add the mushrooms to another pan with a teaspoon of oil and cook over a medium-high heat for about 10 minutes until golden brown and tender. Set aside on a plate, then add the tomatoes and cook for about 3 minutes until soft and slightly golden. Add them to the plate with the mushrooms.

3   When the sausages are nearly ready, crack your eggs into the pan to gently fry. (Feel free to poach or scramble your eggs.) Pop the beans in the microwave for a minute to reheat and add your bread to the toaster. Gently reheat the mushrooms and tomatoes in the pan as well.

4   Once all the elements are ready, plate up and enjoy! No need for ketchup, use the beans and egg yolk for sauce.

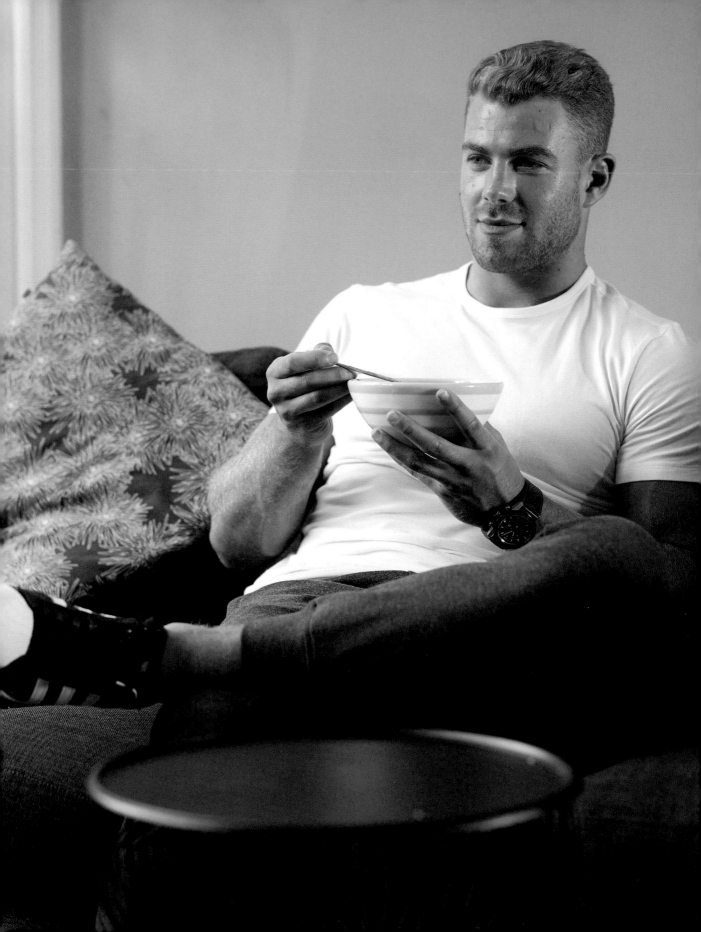

LUNCH & SNACKS

A well-balanced lunch should keep your energy levels up and hunger at bay, so you're not feeling unbearably hungry by 4 o'clock.

All of these lunch recipes can be prepared the night before and reheated the next day, making them super-convenient for any busy lifestyle. I've also included some of my favourite healthy savoury snacks.

CHICKEN SATAY STIR-FRY

I wanted to make my own version of the nation's favourite Chinese dish, chicken satay. For me, this dish proves that healthy food can also be delicious (and vice versa!)

2–3 tsp coconut oil
1 small onion, peeled and diced
1 orange, yellow or red pepper, chopped
½ courgette, sliced
120g quinoa
2 chicken breasts, sliced into chunks
sea salt and freshly ground black pepper

FOR THE SATAY SAUCE
1 tsp crunchy peanut butter (or other nut butter)
1 tsp honey
juice of ½ lime

1   Add the coconut oil to a large frying pan with the onion and cook for 5 minutes over a medium heat. Add the rest of your veg to the pan and increase the heat to medium-high. I like my veg to still have a crunch to it, so stir for about 7–10 minutes.

2   In the meantime, add your quinoa to a pan of boiling water and cook for about 15 minutes.

3   Remove the vegetables from the pan. Add the chicken breast, season and cook until brown, then turn down the heat.

4   Add the nut butter and honey to the pan and, over a low heat, coat the chicken, stirring to combine for about 1 minute, then remove from the heat.

5   Drain the quinoa well and toss with your vegetables. Pour over the silky and sticky satay chicken, squeeze over your fresh lime and tuck in.

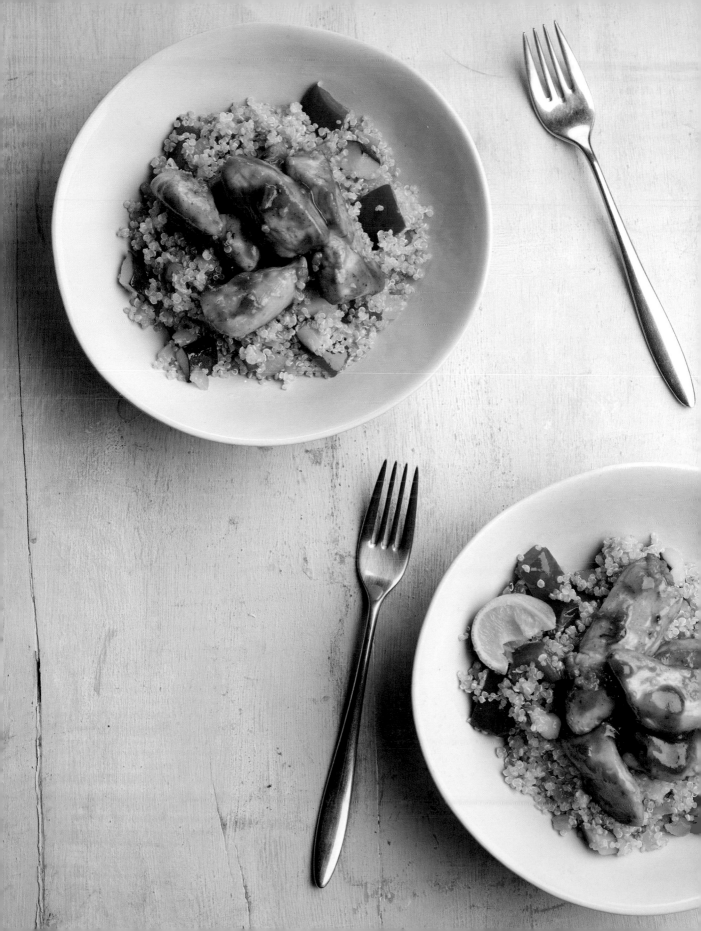

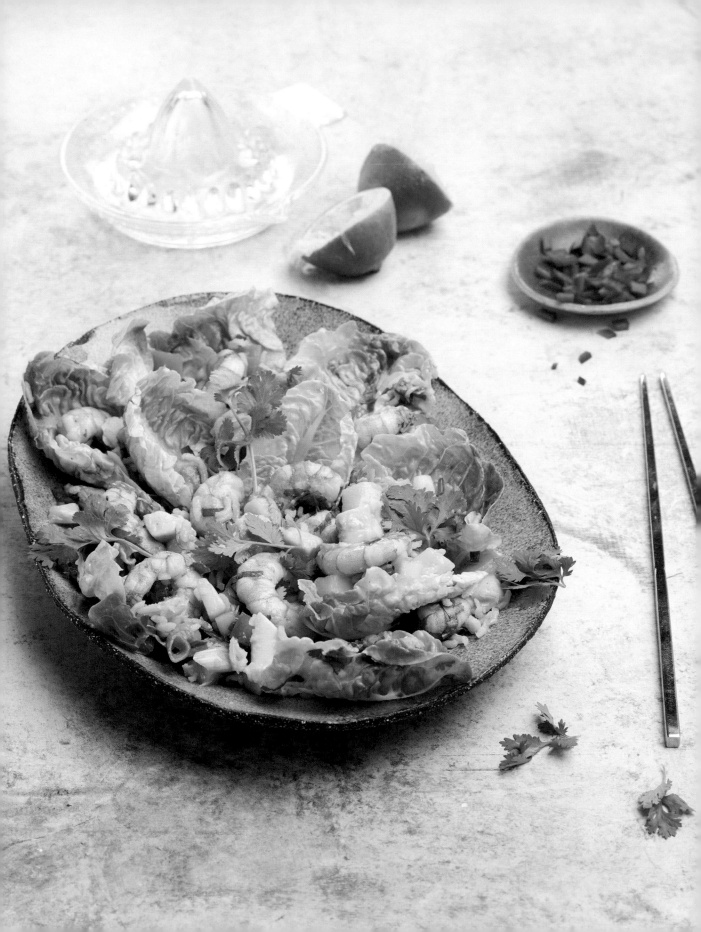

ASIAN-STYLE KING PRAWN AND MANGO SALAD

Fruit doesn't have to be restricted to desserts or snacks. I added mango to this delicious, aromatic and refreshing salad to give it a burst of flavour.

40g wholegrain rice, rinsed, or
   100g cooked wholegrain rice
½ ripe avocado
¼ mango, peeled and diced into
   small cubes
½ red, yellow or orange pepper,
   chopped
1 spring onion, chopped
4 large lettuce leaves, shredded
100g cooked king prawns

FOR THE DRESSING

zest of 1 lime
juice of ½ lime
20g coriander, finely chopped
1 red chilli, deseeded and finely
   chopped
1 heaped tsp honey
1 tsp low-salt soy sauce

1 If using uncooked rice, place the rice in a saucepan and cover with cold water. Bring up to the boil, then cover the pan and simmer over a gentle heat for 20–25 minutes.

2 Whilst the rice cooks, prep the salad. Peel, stone and dice the avocado into small cubes and add to a bowl with your mango, pepper, spring onion and lettuce, tossing together.

3 In a separate bowl, add all of the salad dressing ingredients and stir, then add the prawns and mix until they are all coated in the dressing.

4 Drain the wholegrain rice, leave to cool slightly, then add to the tossed salad followed by the sweet and zingy prawns and toss again before serving.

CREAMY CHICKEN AND PESTO BUCKWHEAT SPAGHETTI

If you're craving some Italian cuisine, this is the dish for you. Creamy pesto and succulent chicken with buckwheat spaghetti. Dig in!

2–3 tsp coconut oil
400g chicken breast, thinly
    sliced
100g buckwheat noodles
basil leaves, to garnish
sea salt and freshly ground black
    pepper

FOR THE PESTO
½ ripe avocado
1 garlic clove, peeled
10 basil leaves
25g spinach
olive oil (optional)

1 Add the coconut oil to a large non-stick pan over a medium heat and chuck in the chicken, season and cook for 5–7 minutes, until golden and cooked through, tossing regularly.

2 Whilst the chicken is frying, add the buckwheat noodles into a pan of boiling water. Simmer for about 5–6 minutes, until tender.

3 Whilst the chicken and the noodles cook, prepare your pesto. Peel and stone the avocado and add with all the other ingredients to a blender with a big pinch of salt. Blitz until smooth and creamy, adding a touch of olive oil if necessary.

4 Turn down the chicken and make sure it is not sticking to the pan. Drain the noodles, saving 2 tablespoons of the water.

5 Add the noodles to the chicken and then the pesto and stir until everything is completed coated in the pesto sauce, adding the reserved 2 tablespoons of water to loosen. Garnish with a few basil leaves and serve.

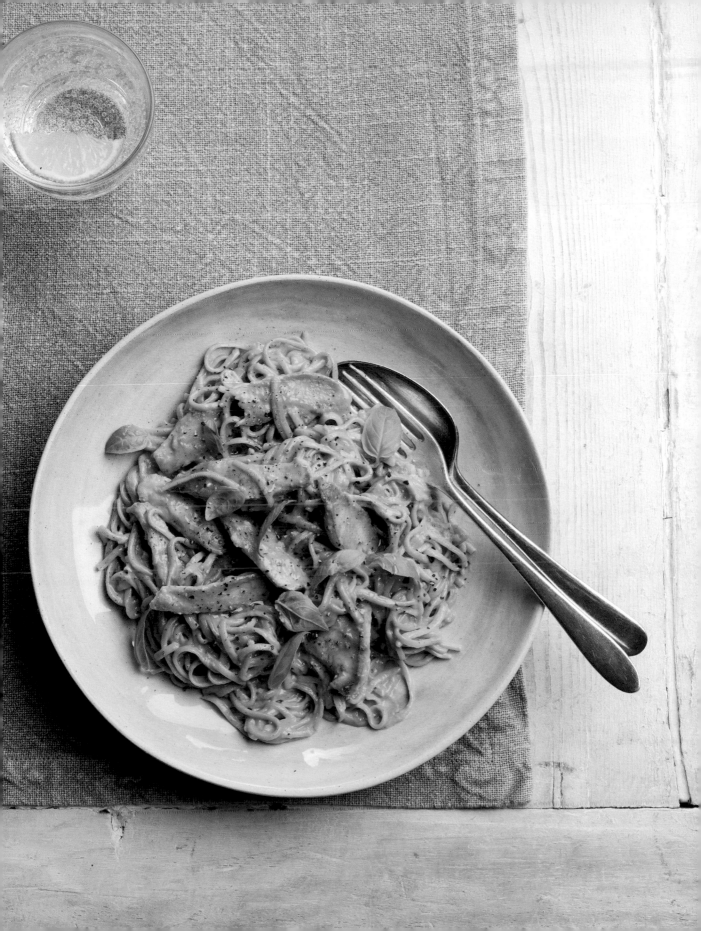

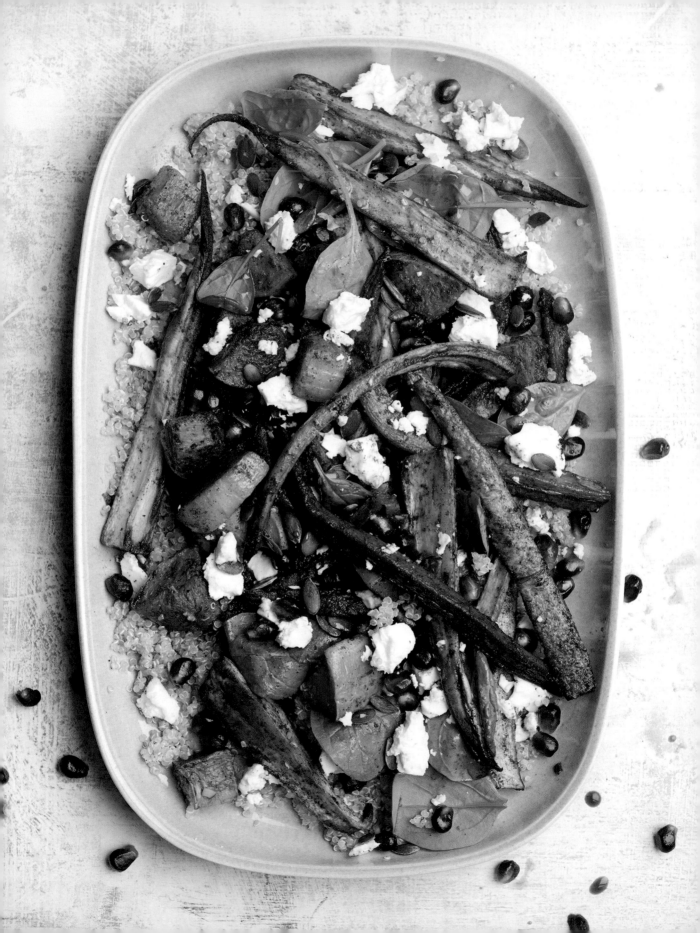

SPICED ROASTED ROOT VEGETABLES WITH FETA AND POMEGRANATE

Veggies will love this dish; it's bursting with flavour and fills you right up after a workout.

½ butternut squash, peeled and
cubed (about 500g)
4 carrots, peeled and sliced
lengthways
2 parsnips, peeled and sliced
lengthways
150g peeled sweet potato, cubed
2 tbsp olive oil
160g quinoa, rinsed
juice of ½ lemon
60g bag of spinach
30g feta cheese
generous handful of pomegranate
seeds
20g pumpkin seeds
sea salt and freshly ground black
pepper

FOR THE SPICES
½ tsp ground cinnamon
1 tsp ground cumin
1 tsp ground ginger
½ tsp paprika
½ tsp ground turmeric
¼ tsp cayenne

1 Preheat the oven to 200°C/180°C fan/gas 6.

2 Mix all the spices together with a pinch of salt to create a Moroccan-style blend.

3 Add the sliced and cubed root vegetables to a roasting dish, season with the spice mix, drizzle over the olive oil and toss so everything is covered evenly. Add to the oven and roast for 45 minutes, tossing the vegetables after 25 minutes.

4 Whilst the root vegetables roast, cook the quinoa in a pan of boiling water for about 15 minutes.

5 Once cooked, drain thoroughly, squeeze over the lemon juice and season with a pinch of salt and pepper.

6 Plate up the quinoa, top it with the spicy root vegetables and then sprinkle over the spinach leaves, feta, pomegranate seeds and pumpkin seeds for a pop of flavour, crunch and creaminess.

MY BEST BEETROOT AND RED PEPPER SALAD WITH WALNUTS AND GOAT'S CHEESE

This is a simple and delicious salad, which is easy to prepare and doesn't sacrifice any flavour or food groups. It's great to take to the office as you can pre-prep all the ingredients in bulk on a Sunday, bring them into work on a Monday and store everything in the fridge ready to assemble in the proportions you like for the next few days.

½ small sweet potato, peeled and chopped into 1cm cubes (about 100g)
100g cooked beetroot, chopped
1 red pepper, diced
big handful of mixed salad leaves
5 walnuts, crushed or finely chopped
40g crumbly goat's cheese or feta cheese

FOR THE DRESSING
1 tbsp olive oil
2 tsp balsamic vinegar
sea salt and freshly ground black pepper

1   Preheat the oven to 200°C/180°C fan/gas 6.

2   Bake the sweet potato for 25–30 minutes or boil for 15 minutes. If this salad is for work, always have cooked sweet potato readily available in your fridge, it's still really good reheated.

3   Once the sweet potato is cooked, add all the ingredients to a bowl and toss together.

4   Mix the olive oil and vinegar together with some seasoning and drizzle over the salad.

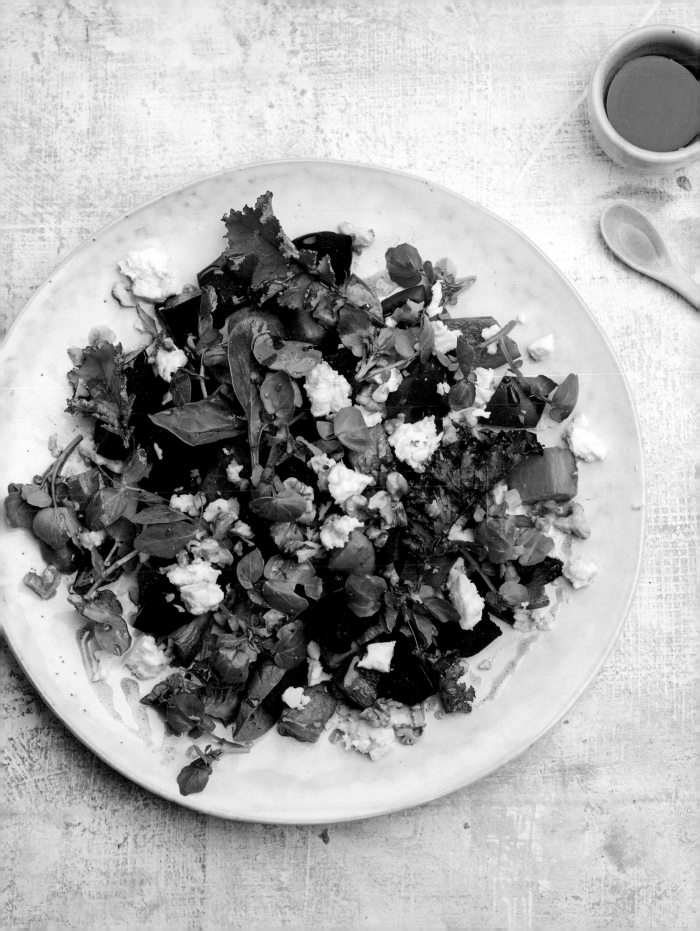

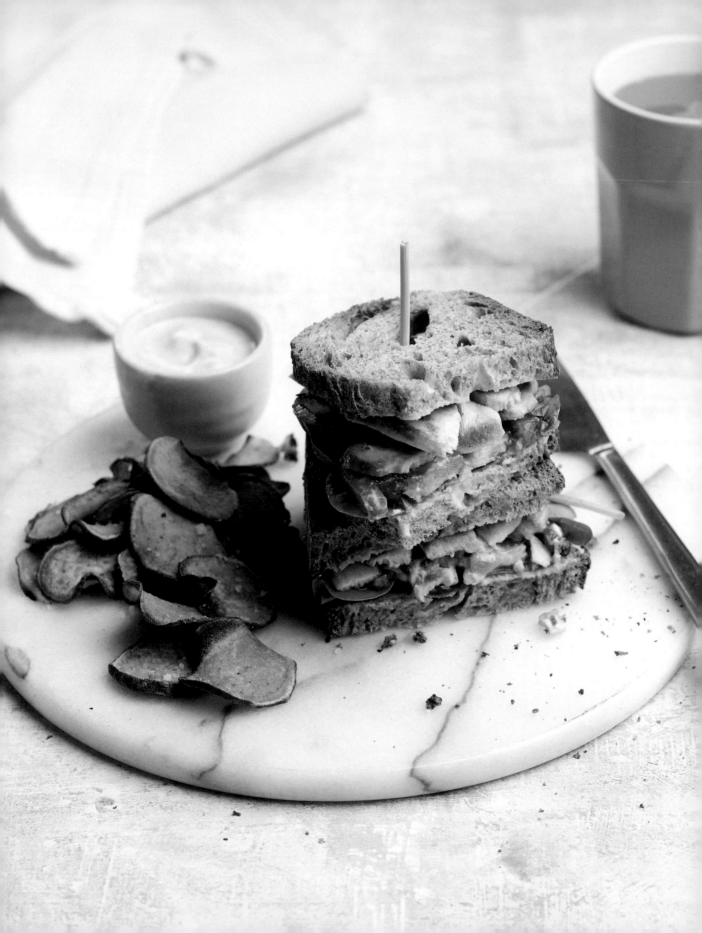

TOASTED SOURDOUGH CLT WITH HOMEMADE CRISPS

If you love a cheeky sandwich meal deal, move away from the supermarket fridge and give this bad boy a go.

1 chicken breast, thinly sliced
1 tsp coconut oil
2 slices of sourdough or rye
   bread, toasted
½ tbsp crème fraîche
½ tsp Dijon or English mustard
½ beef tomato, sliced
small handful of spinach leaves

FOR THE HOMEMADE CRISPS
1 small sweet potato, thinly
   sliced (about 150g)
drizzle of olive oil
sea salt and freshly ground black
   pepper

1   Preheat the oven to 220°C/200°C fan/gas 7.

2   Lay the slices of sweet potato onto a baking tray, drizzle with olive oil and season. Toss to fully coat. These should only need 10–15 minutes to bake, but keep an eye on them. Turn them halfway through the cooking time. You want them to start getting brown around the edges and crisp up.

3   In the meantime, cook the thinly sliced chicken breast in a touch of oil for about 5 minutes, tossing until golden and cooked through.

4   Add the bread to the toaster and make sure it is nice and crunchy.

5   Mix the crème fraîche with the mustard and spread on each side of the bread.

6   Layer on the tomato, spinach leaves and chicken and cut in half.

7   Remove the sweet potato crisps and let them cool down. Add extra seasoning to taste and serve with the sandwich.

FILLET STEAK WITH CHILLI BROCCOLI AND COURGETTE AND SWEET POTATO FRIES

Splash the cash and jazz things up with this steak lunch. I try to treat myself once a week to a good-quality fillet steak.

1 large courgette, chopped into finger-sized chunks
1 sweet potato, unpeeled and chopped into finger-sized chunks (about 200g)
2 drizzles of olive oil
150g tenderstem broccoli
1 fillet steak (about 300g)
1 tbsp coconut oil
pinch of chilli flakes
sea salt and freshly ground black pepper

1   Preheat the oven to 220°C/200°C fan/gas 7.

2   Add the courgette and sweet potato to a baking tray, season with salt and pepper and drizzle with olive oil. Put in the middle of the oven to bake for 20–25 minutes, tossing halfway through.

3   Meanwhille, add the broccoli to a steamer or a saucepan of boiling water and steam or simmer for around 7 minutes, until tender.

4   Season your steak and add the coconut oil to a non-stick frying pan. Make sure the oil and pan are hot before you add the steak. Cook the steak for as long as you like it, turning it once. I'd say a 2cm-thick steak would be 4 minutes each side for medium.

5   Drain the broccoli and place back into the pan without the water. Coat in a drizzle of olive oil and sprinkle over the chilli flakes – leave over a low heat for a minute.

6   Remove the steak from the pan and let it rest for a few minutes. Once rested, slice into strips.

7   Now plate up the broccoli, sweet potato and courgette on a plate next to your juicy, tender steak.

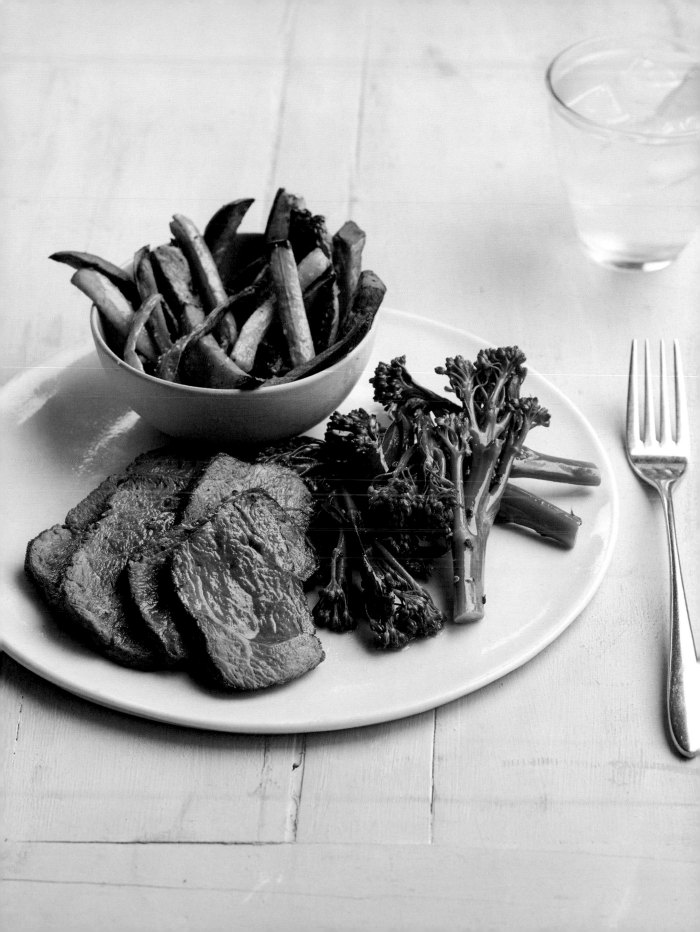

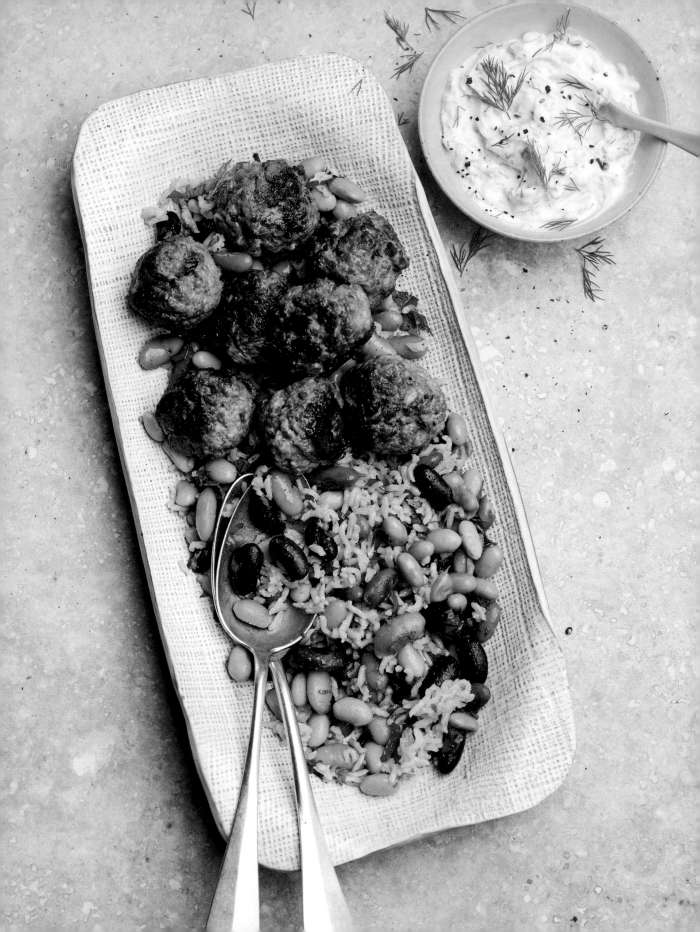

LEAN TURKEY MEATBALLS WITH MIXED BEAN AND EDAMAME SALAD

We used to have spaghetti and meatballs a lot and I love them, so I created this super-lean recipe to feed my cravings.

FOR THE MEATBALLS

250g lean minced turkey
2 spring onions, trimmed and finely
    chopped
2 tbsp Parmesan cheese
½ tsp paprika
1 tbsp coconut oil
sea salt and freshly ground black pepper

FOR THE BEAN SALAD

30g wholegrain rice, rinsed, or 75g
    cooked wholegrain rice
1 x 400g tin of mixed bean salad,
    drained and rinsed
30g edamame beans
2 tbsp apple cider vinegar
1 tbsp olive oil
½ tsp ground cumin
1 tbsp chopped parsley

FOR THE TZATZIKI

3 heaped tbsp Greek yoghurt
6cm piece of cucumber, cut in half,
    deseeded, grated and drained
½ garlic clove, peeled and crushed
small grating of lemon zest
squeeze of lemon juice
small handful of chopped parsley

1   If using uncooked rice, place the rice in a saucepan and cover with cold water. Bring up to the boil, then cover the pan and simmer over a gentle heat for 20–25 minutes.

2   Add all the meatball ingredients (except the coconut oil) to a bowl and mix together well. I prefer to use my hands, making sure they are very clean. Season with salt and a big pinch of pepper.

3   Roll into eight golf ball-sized amounts and add to a hot large frying pan with the coconut oil. Fry over a medium-high heat for 7–10 minutes, until completely cooked through.

4   Meanwile, make the bean salad and tzatziki. For the bean salad, simply add all the ingredients to a bowl and stir, adding the wholegrain rice once cooked. For the tzatziki, again simply add all the ingredients to a bowl with a pinch of sea salt and freshly ground black pepper and stir.

5   Once the meatballs are brown on the outside, check the inside of one to ensure it is cooked through.

6   Plate up the bean salad and rice and top it with four meatballs and a dollop of tzatziki.

SPICY SALMON FISH CAKE BITES

Sometimes snacking on chicken can get boring. I love salmon and these little bites are delicious, not to mention convenient.

2 salmon fillets, skinless (or you can use any fish) (about 270g in total)
1 tbsp finely chopped coriander
1 chilli, deseeded and finely chopped
juice and zest of ½ lime
1 shallot or ½ small red onion, finely chopped
1 large egg
1 tsp coconut oil
sea salt and freshly ground black pepper

1   Put the fish in a food processor or blender and mince, but not too much.

2   Add to a bowl with the coriander, chilli, lime juice and zest and onion and mix together.

3   Mix in the egg and season with salt and pepper.

4   Melt the coconut oil in a frying pan and then add heaped spoonfuls of the mixture, around 6cm in diameter, to the pan. Cook over a medium-high heat for 5–6 minutes, flipping them halfway through, until golden and cooked through.

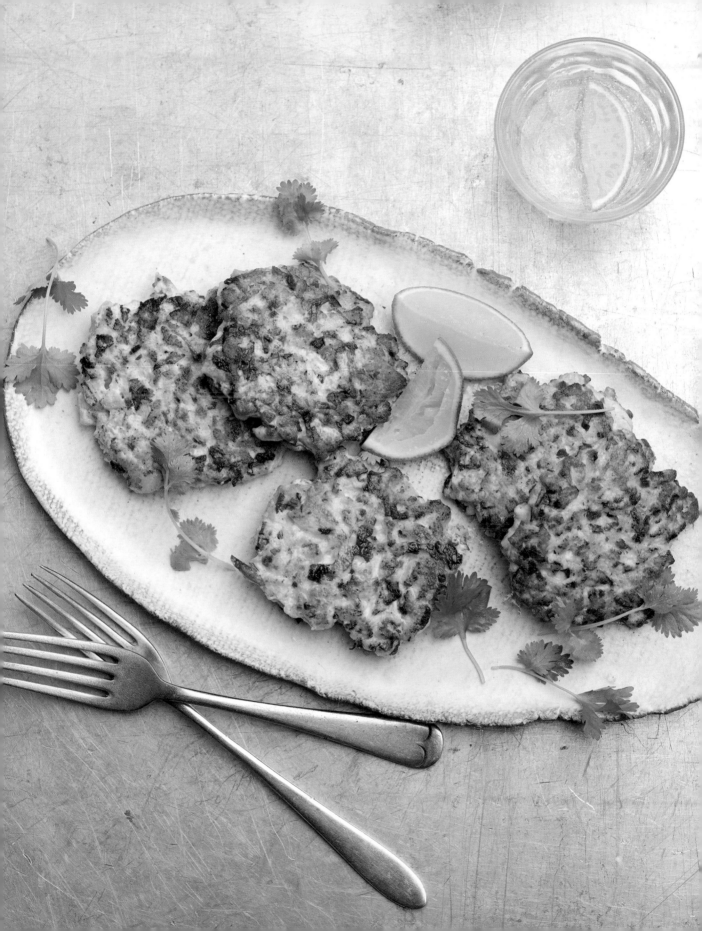

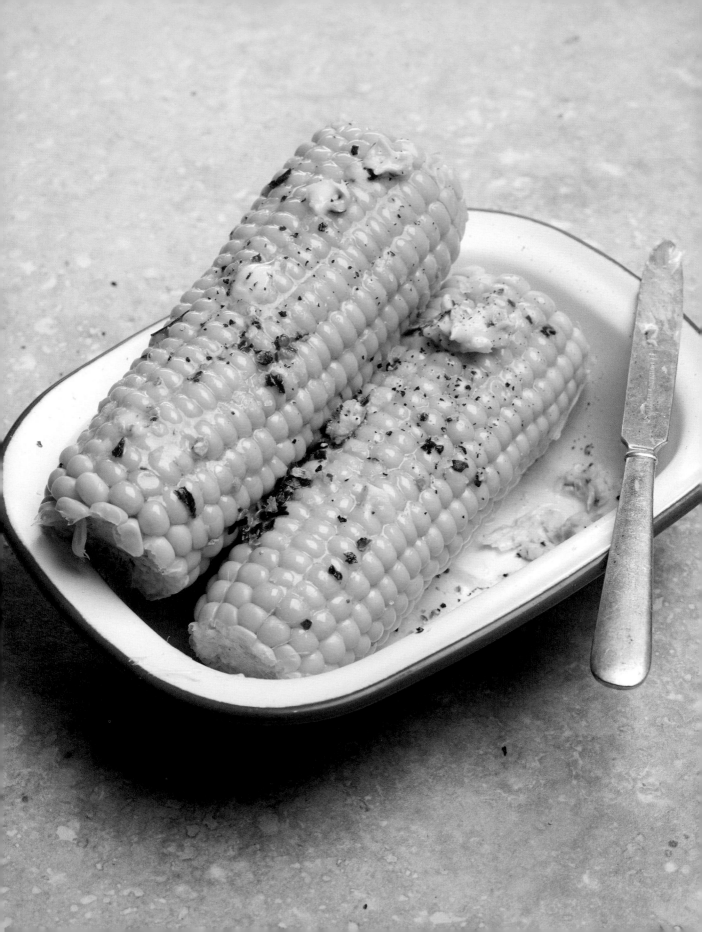

CORN ON THE COB WITH CHILLI BUTTER

This is super-simple and makes a great savoury snack that can curb a craving for the sweet stuff.

2 corn on the cob
½ tsp chilli flakes
2 tsp unsalted butter, softened
sea salt and freshly ground black
   pepper

1   Add the cobs to a pan of boiling water and let it boil for about 7 minutes.

2   Mix the chilli flakes in with the butter and brush onto the sweetcorn.

3   Sprinkle salt and pepper all the way around. Get your teeth stuck into that.

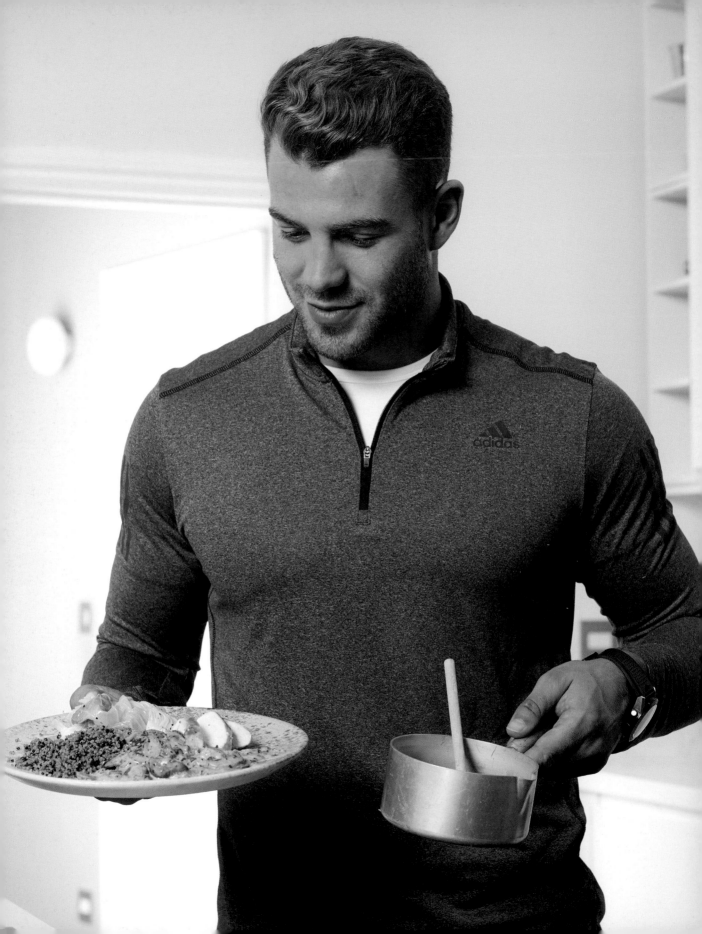

DINNER

I never go to bed with a rumbling stomach; nor do I like to go to bed with a belly full of food.

For me dinner should be the lightest meal of the day; unless I've gone to the gym in the evening then I'll have a little more on my plate.

SWEET-AND-SPICY ASIAN SALMON WITH PAK CHOI

This is one of my signature dishes – it's full of flavour but so simple to make. It is one of the meals I really look forward to eating and crave the most.

50g wholegrain rice, rinsed, or
    125g cooked wholegrain rice
1 pak choi bulb, washed and
    sliced lengthways into wedges
2 tsp coconut oil
1 large salmon fillet (about 140g)

FOR THE DRESSING
2 tsp honey
2 tbsp tamari or low-salt soy sauce
big pinch of chilli flakes or
    chopped fresh chilli
2–3cm piece of fresh ginger, finely
    chopped, or 1 tsp ginger purée
1 garlic clove, peeled and crushed

1 If using uncooked rice, place the rice in a saucepan and cover with cold water. Bring up to the boil, then cover the pan and simmer over a gentle heat for 20–25 minutes.

2 Steam your pak choi for about 6 minutes, until tender. Either pour boiling water halfway up a saucepan and top it with a colander or steamer, placing the pak choi into the colander with a lid on top or, if you have a steamer, follow the instructions.

3 Make your dressing by stirring all of the ingredients together in a bowl. Let the flavours infuse.

4 Add the coconut oil to a frying pan over a high heat. Once melted, place the salmon fillet into the pan skin side down. Hold it there for a few moments so it doesn't curl up.

5 Gently turn the salmon over; it should only need 3 minutes each side to get it just cooked through. In the last minute, pour over the dressing you've just made. It will sizzle, so reduce the heat to medium-low for the final 30 seconds or so.

6 Now plate everything up, ensuring you drizzle what is left of the sauce all over the dish

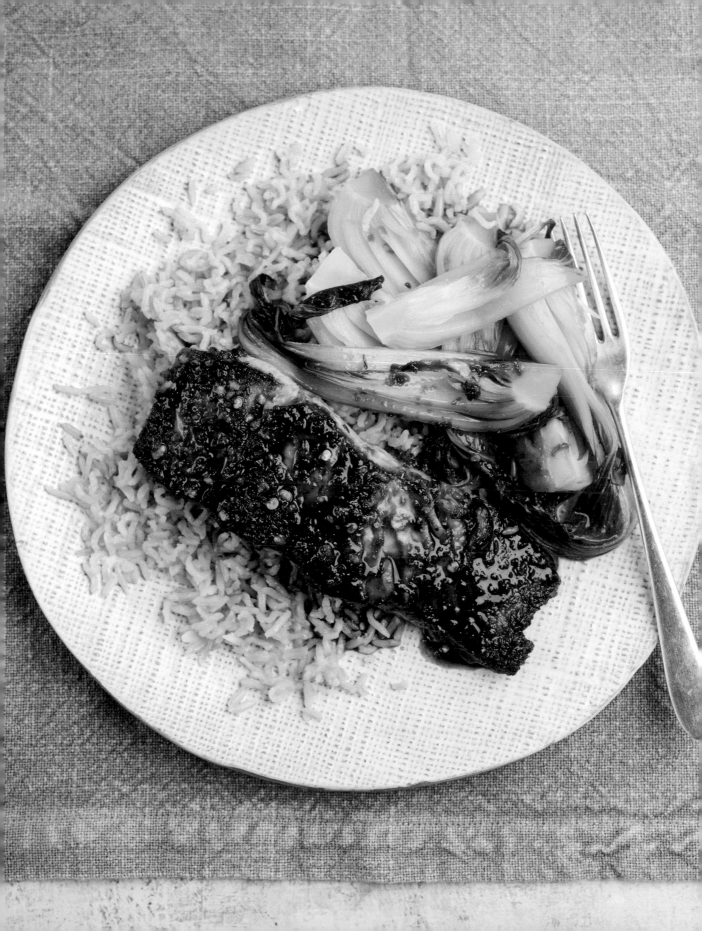

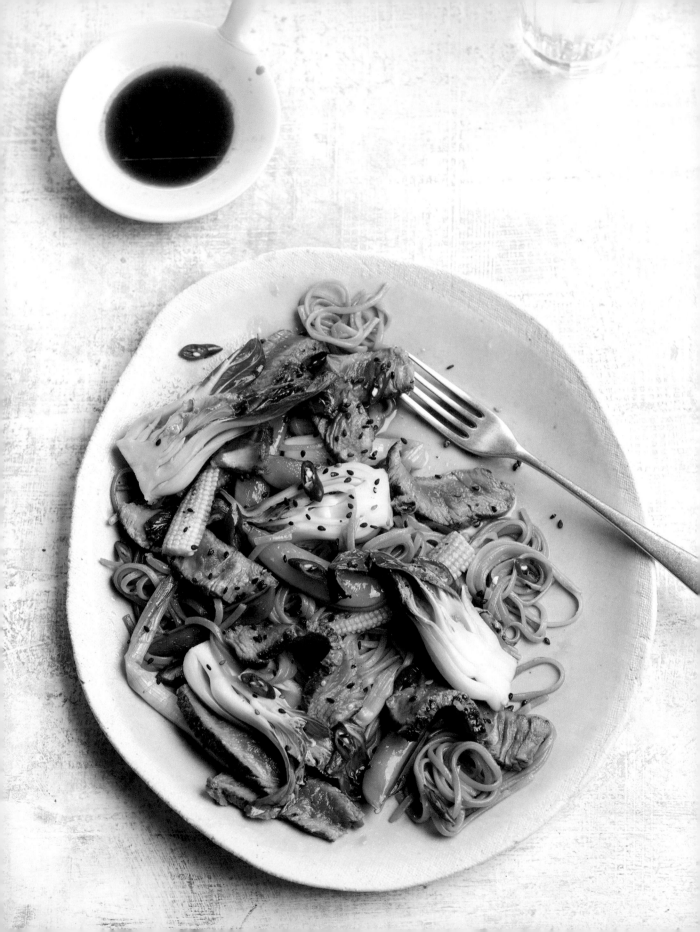

BEEF IT UP TERIYAKI STIR-FRY

If I've gone a week without red meat I love to tuck into this beefy stir-fry. Feel free to swap the beef with chicken, salmon, tofu or prawns if you prefer. Please feel free to add extra vegetables to the dish too.

120g buckwheat noodles

1 tbsp coconut oil

300–400g lean frying steak or flat-iron steak

1 packet of stir-fry vegetables (mine was 400g)

sea salt and freshly ground black pepper

½ tbsp sesame seeds, to serve (optional)

FOR THE TERIYAKI SAUCE

3½ tbsp tamari or low-salt soy sauce

2 tbsp honey

2–3cm piece of fresh ginger, finely chopped or grated

1 garlic clove, peeled and finely chopped, or 1 tsp ginger purée

1 tsp sesame oil

2 tbsp mirin or sake (optional)

1 Start by making the teriyaki sauce. Add all of the ingredients to a small saucepan and put over a medium-high heat. Bring to the boil, then reduce the heat and simmer gently for 2–3 minutes, until slightly thickened. Set aside.

2 Add the noodles to a pan of boiling water and cook for about 6 minutes.

3 In the meantime, add the coconut oil to a hot wok. When melted, add the beef to the pan and season with salt and pepper. Stir-fry for around 2 minutes over a high heat, then remove from the pan and set aside.

4 Add in the vegetables and stir-fry for about 3–4 minutes. Drain the noodles, saving about a tablespoon of water. Add the noodles to the veg along with the beef and all its juices and toss around so they are all evenly distributed. Now pour over the teriyaki sauce and cook for a further minute, stirring so everything is coated in the silky sauce. If you want extra sauce, add the water from the noodles. Sprinkle over the sesame seeds, if using, to serve.

POST-WORKOUT PIRI-PIRI CHICKEN PLATE

The perfect protein-packed plate after a workout – or at any time of the day really. It's a definite favourite of mine.

2 sweet potatoes (about 350g in total)
olive oil, for cooking
2 large chicken breasts (about 200g each), thickly sliced
juice of ½ lemon
½ ripe avocado
½ bag of mixed salad leaves (50g in total)
10 cherry tomatoes, halved
2 corn on the cobs
2 tbsp Greek yoghurt
1 tbsp mixed seeds

FOR THE PIRI-PIRI SEASONING RUB
½ tsp paprika
1 tsp dried oregano, crushed
1 tsp ground ginger
½ tsp ground cardamom
1 tsp garlic powder
1 tsp onion powder/granules
½ tsp salt
½ tsp ground piri-piri pepper (or ¼ tsp cayenne pepper)

1   Preheat the oven to 220°C/200°C fan/gas 7.

2   Mix all the spices together in a bowl to create your piri-piri seasoning rub.

3   Slice the sweet potatoes into skinny wedges and place on a baking tray with a drizzle (around ½ tablespoon) of olive oil and a sprinkle of the piri-piri seasoning. Bake for 30 minutes, tossing halfway through.

4   Meanwhile, prepare the chicken. Put the remainder of the seasoning into a sandwich bag or toss in a bowl with the chicken and shake so the chicken is completely covered. Place on a large sheet of foil, squeeze over the lemon and a drizzle of oil, then fold the foil over and seal the edges to create a parcel. Place this into the oven to bake for 20–25 minutes.

5   Peel and stone the avocado and chop into chunks. Put the salad leaves, tomatoes and avocado into a bowl and toss.

6   Add the corn cobs to a saucepan of boiling water and boil for about 6 minutes.

7   Once your chicken, potatoes and corn are done, add a tablespoon of Greek yoghurt to your plate, sprinkle with seeds and use for dipping your wedges in. Enjoy the succulent piri-piri chicken and sides.

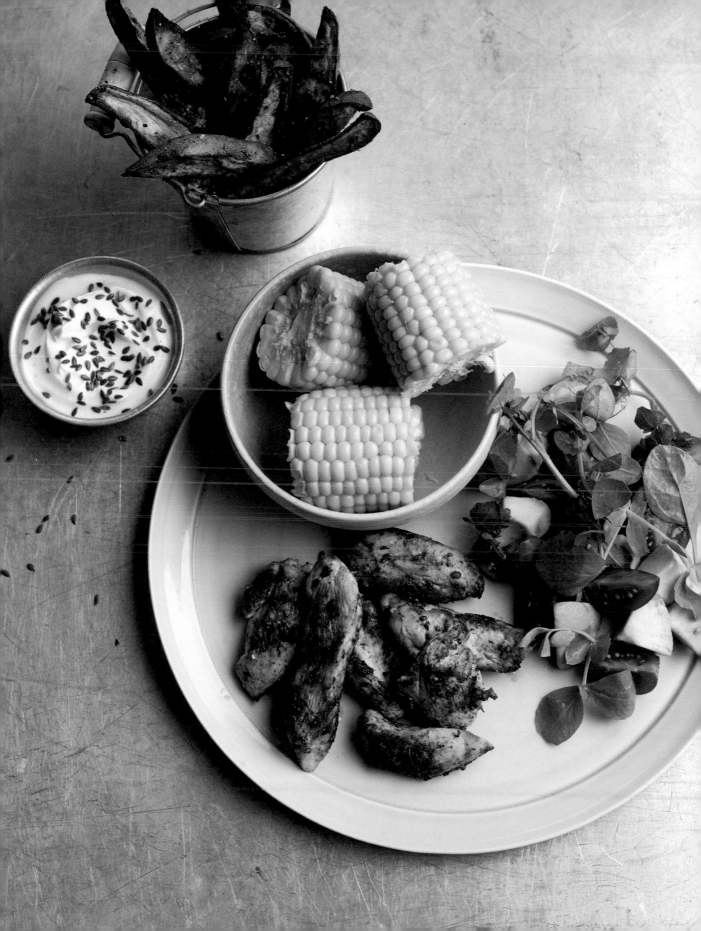

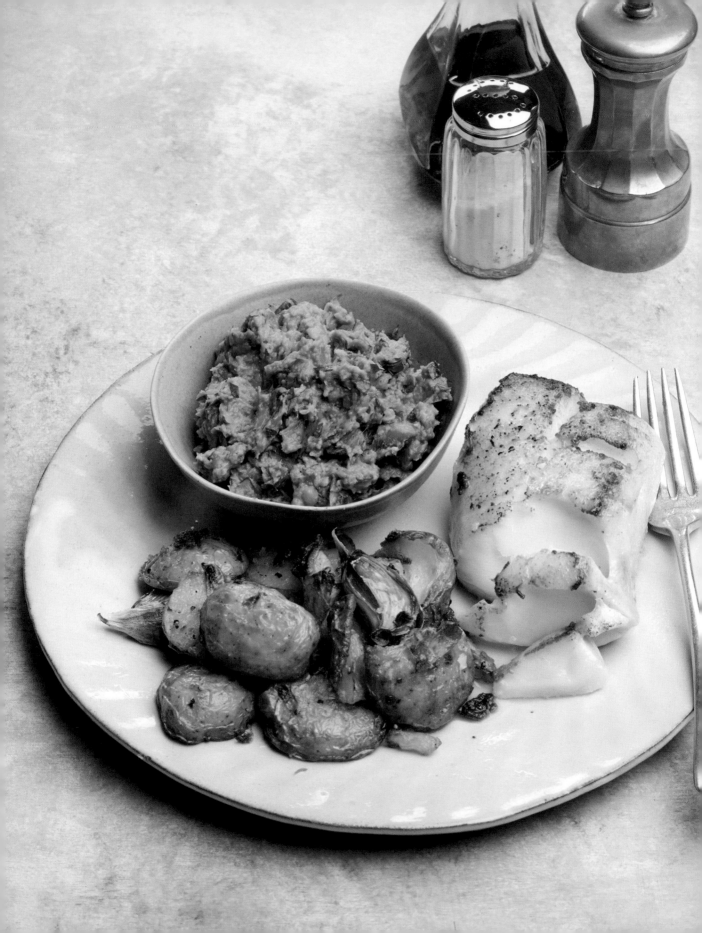

FISH, CRISPY POTATOES AND MUSHY PEAS

There is nothing like fish and chips on a Friday, and eating healthily shouldn't mean missing out on your favourite traditions!

300g new potatoes, halved
1½ tbsp olive oil
1 unpeeled garlic clove, bashed
2 large white fish fillets, skin on preferably (mine was skin off, but it is so delicate when pan-fried) (175–200g each)
splash of apple cider vinegar

FOR THE MUSHY PEAS
75g frozen petits pois
100g asparagus, chopped into 2cm chunks
¼ small onion, peeled and diced
½ tbsp olive oil
½ tbsp parsley leaves
sea salt and freshly ground black pepper

1   Begin by adding the new potatoes to a pan of boiling water. Boil for 15–20 minutes or until tender.

2   In the meantime, add the olive oil to a large frying pan and fry the peas, asparagus, onion and a pinch of salt and pepper over a medium-high heat for 5 minutes, then add a tablespoon of water and cover with a lid. Reduce the heat to medium-low, leaving it for a further 3–5 minutes.

3   Once cooked, add to a blender with the parsley and blitz up until smooth but still slightly lumpy for that mushy pea texture. Keep aside whilst you prepare the rest of the dish. You can also do this with a stick blender.

4   Drain the new potatoes, then return them to the pan. Squash each potato with a fork and drizzle in ½ tablespoon of the olive oil and the bashed garlic. Turn up the heat and watch them go all crunchy around the edges.

5   Finally, add the remaining tablespoon of olive oil to a non-stick pan and place the fillets in, seasoning them on both sides, and fry over a high heat for about 3–4 minutes in total, flipping halfway through.

6   Remove the fish and add to your plate with the mushy peas and crunchy new potatoes. Season with salt and vinegar and enjoy.

STEAK WITH GARLIC AND PARMESAN MUSHROOMS AND VEGETABLE MASH

This is a great dinner for two on a Friday night in, without all the bloating and guilt that a greasy take-away brings.

4 tsp good-quality unsalted butter, softened

½ tbsp finely chopped parsley

1 small garlic clove, peeled and crushed

1 tbsp grated Parmesan

6 chestnut mushrooms, stalks removed

1 tbsp olive oil

2 fillet or sirloin steaks (about 300g each)

sea salt and freshly ground black pepper

FOR THE ROOT VEGETABLES (CHOOSE 600G OF ANY MIX, SUCH AS)

1 sweet potato, peeled and sliced into 2cm chunks

2 carrots, peeled and sliced into 2cm chunks

1 parsnip, peeled and sliced into 2cm chunks

½ swede, peeled and sliced into 2cm chunks

1 Preheat the oven to 200°C/180°C fan/gas 6.

2 In a bowl, mix 2 teaspoons of the butter, the parsley, crushed garlic and Parmesan and evenly distribute into the hole of each mushroom. Place the mushrooms onto a baking tray and put in the centre of the oven to bake for about 15 minutes.

3 Cook all the vegetables in a large saucepan of boiling water for about 20 minutes or until completely tender.

4 Whilst the vegetables and mushrooms are cooking, pour the olive oil into a frying pan over a high heat and add the seasoned steaks. For a medium finish, cook for 4 minutes each side. Remove the steaks and let rest on a chopping board or plate for 5 minutes, then slice.

5 Drain the root vegetables thoroughly and then add the rest of the butter, salt and pepper and mash until as smooth as possible.

6 Now remove the mushrooms from the oven and plate up all the elements. Not bad if you ask me.

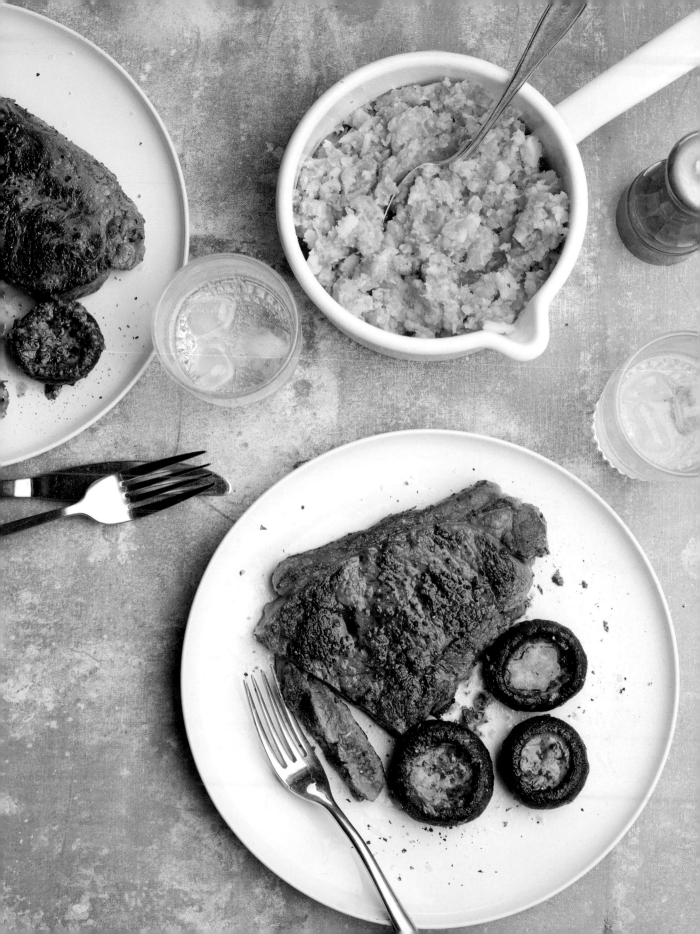

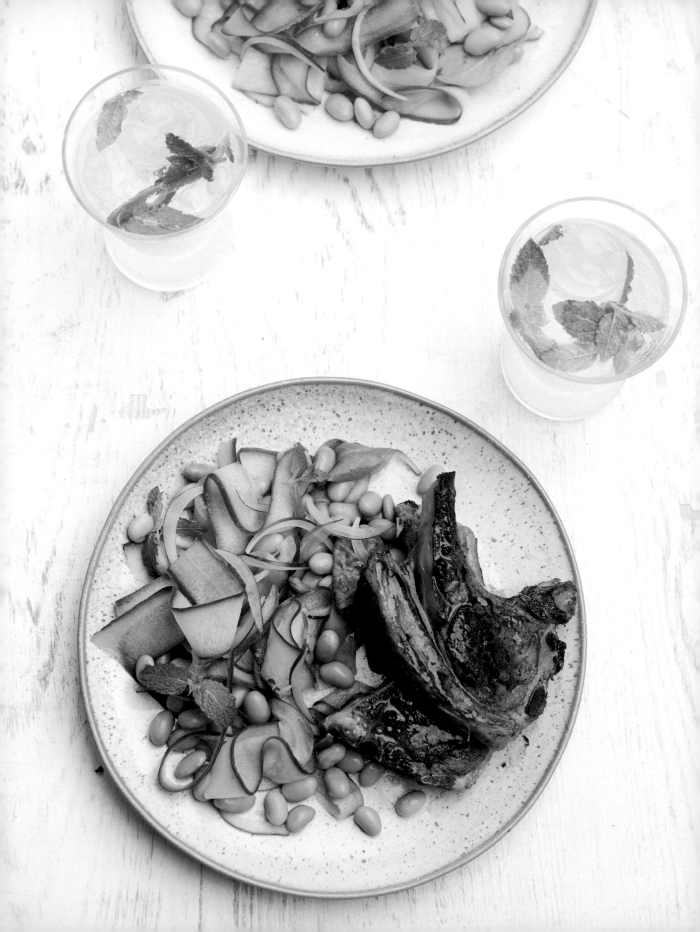

MINT LAMB WITH SUPER GREEN SALAD

This is such a light, fresh dish. I enjoy it most on a Sunday in the sunshine.

2 tbsp olive oil

1 tbsp honey

1 tbsp fresh mint leaves, finely chopped

1 tsp dried mint

1 tsp apple cider vinegar

4 lamb chops or lamb leg steaks

½ cucumber, peeled into ribbons with a vegetable peeler

1 x 400g tin of mixed beans or butter beans, drained and rinsed (optional)

100g edamame beans

60g bag of baby spinach

½ red onion, peeled and thinly sliced

juice of ½ lemon

sea salt and freshly ground black pepper

1   Start by making the mint marinade for the lamb (if you can do this the night before and let them marinate overnight, even better). Add the olive oil, honey, fresh mint, dried mint and cider vinegar to a bowl and stir well to combine. Pour all over the lamb and massage it into the meat.

2   Place the lamb either on a preheated barbecue, grill or hot chargrill pan. You don't need oil as the lamb is already coated in it. Sprinkle over some salt and pepper to season.

3   Whilst the lamb cooks over a medium-high heat (3–4 minutes each side for a slightly pink finish), prepare the salad.

4   Add the cucumber, beans (if using), edamame, spinach and sliced onion to a bowl with the lemon juice and toss together. Season with salt and pepper and toss again.

5   Plate up the salad in abundance and top with your sweet, refreshing minty lamb.

TUNA STEAK WITH CHUNKY TOMATO SALSA AND AVOCADO SALAD

I love Mediterranean food – the fresh ingredients and simple flavours of this dish take me back to my holidays in Spain, Italy and Greece.

50g wholegrain rice, rinsed, or 125g cooked wholegrain rice

½ avocado

1 beef tomato, cut into chunks

¼ red onion, peeled and thinly sliced

5 black olives, pitted and roughly chopped

small handful of basil leaves, chopped

1 tuna steak (about 120g)

1½ tbsp olive oil

juice of ½ lemon

sea salt and freshly ground black pepper

1   If using uncooked rice, place the rice in a saucepan and cover with cold water. Bring up to the boil, then cover the pan and simmer over a gentle heat for 20–25 minutes.

2   In the meantime, prepare your salad by peeling and removing the stone from the avocado and cutting into chunks. Add the avocado, tomato, red onion, olives and basil to a bowl and toss, trying not to mush up the avocado. We will add the dressing at the end.

3   When the rice is nearly done, brush the tuna steak on each side with 1 tablespoon of the olive oil. Place gently into a hot pan and sear on each side for 1 minute over a high heat. The tuna steak is best served with a pink centre. Season and cut into slices.

4   Now drain the rice and add it to the salad, again gently tossing, but be mindful of the avocado. Plate up the rice salad and top it with the tuna slices.

5   Squeeze over the lemon juice and another drizzle of oil with a pinch of seasoning. Now tuck into the fresh flavours of the Mediterranean.

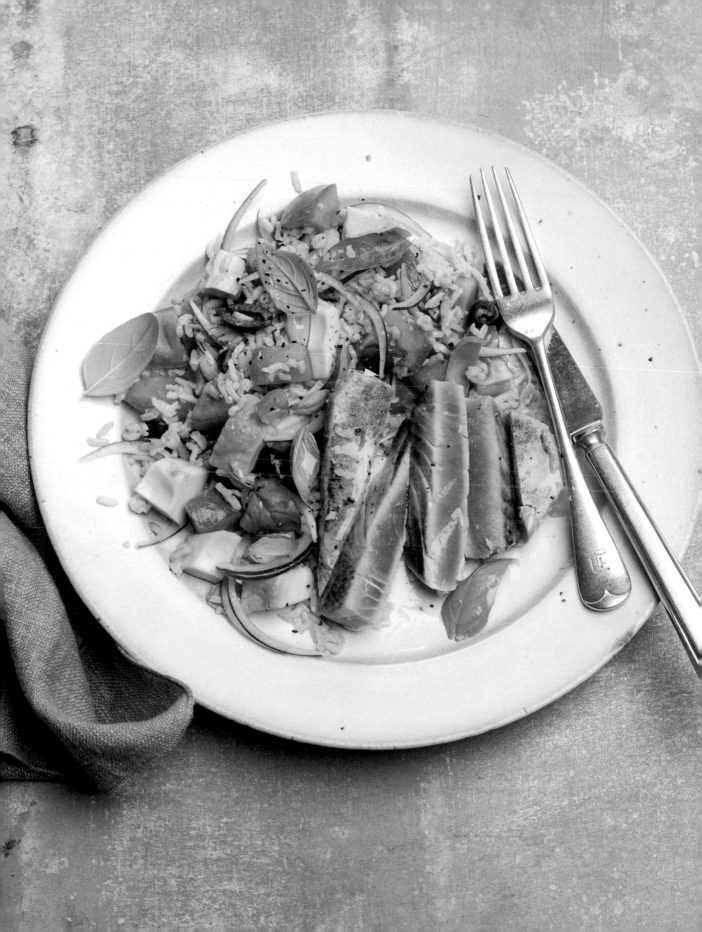

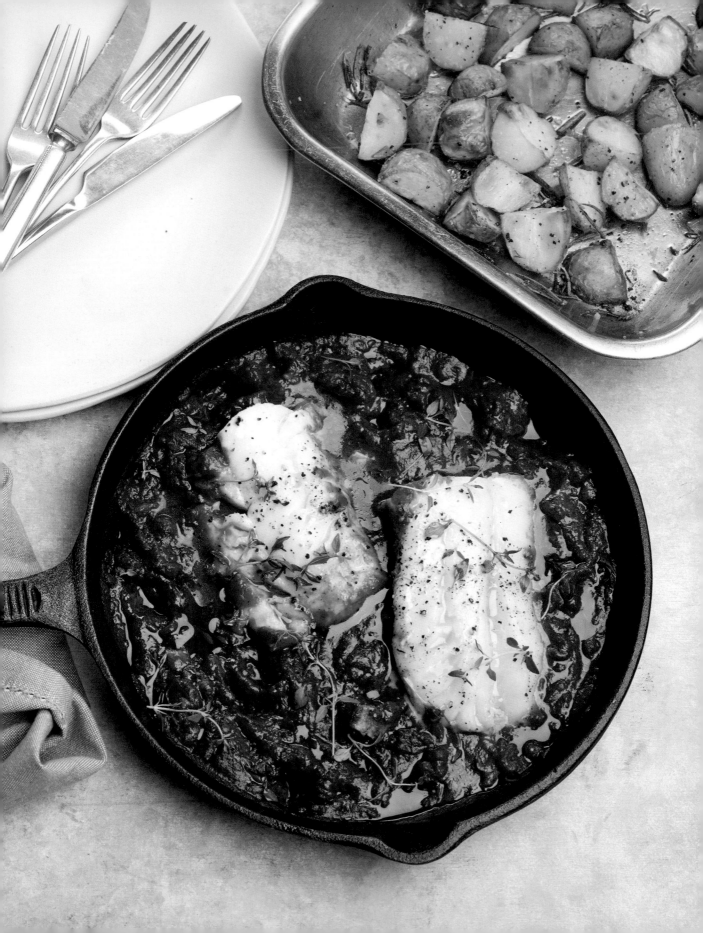

POACHED COD IN A TOMATO AND THYME SAUCE WITH CRUNCHY NEW POTATOES

If you fancy something with a bit of body, but that's still light on your stomach, try this.

300g new potatoes
1 tbsp olive oil
2 sprigs of rosemary, leaves picked
1 x 400g tin chopped tomatoes
½ tbsp tomato purée
200ml vegetable stock
1 garlic clove, peeled and crushed
2 white fish fillets, skin on (about 175g each)
2 sprigs of thyme
100g tenderstem broccoli
sea salt and freshly ground black pepper

1 Preheat the oven to 220°C/200°C fan/gas 7.

2 Cut the new potatoes into quarters so they are nice and small. Place onto a baking tray, drizzle the olive oil all over them and season well. Place just above the middle of the oven and cook for 25–30 minutes, tossing and sprinkling rosemary over halfway through.

3 Add the tin of tomatoes, tomato purée, vegetable stock and garlic to a deep frying pan, stir and let it simmer for 5–7 minutes over a medium heat.

4 Add the cod to the pan, coating with the sauce along with the thyme. Season and let poach in the sauce for a further 10 minutes over a medium-low heat.

5 Boil or steam the broccoli in a separate saucepan for about 7 minutes so it cooks at the same time as the fish.

6 Check the potatoes; they should be golden, then start plating up. Add a fillet of cod to each plate with the crispy rosemary potatoes and a side of broccoli and pour the tomato sauce over.

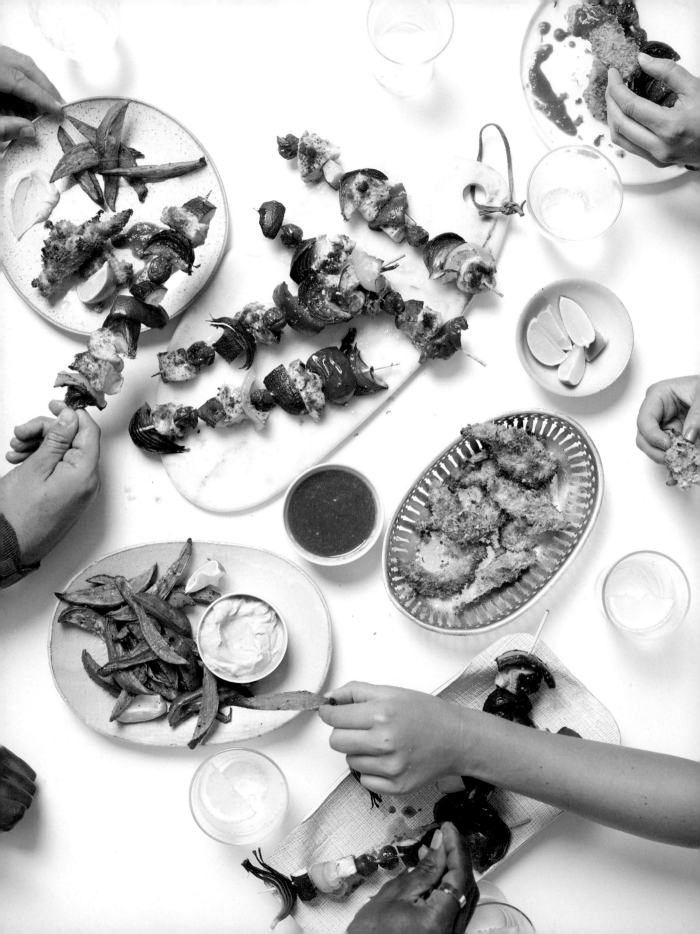

SOCIAL SHARERS

People who love to eat are always the best company.

Just because you're revamping your cooking skills and refreshing your cupboards, doesn't mean the fun is over – if anything it has just begun. Be a good influence and create some deliciously wholesome food for family and friends to enjoy too!

GREEN THAI CHICKEN HOT POT

This is a fuss-free one-pot wonder that's full of that aromatic green Thai flavour we've grown to love.

1 tbsp coconut oil

1 red onion, peeled and chopped

100g wholegrain or basmati rice, rinsed

1 courgette, sliced into 5mm-thick rounds

2 peppers, deseeded and cut into strips

5 tbsp green Thai curry paste

zest and juice of 1 lime

400ml coconut milk

400g chicken breast, cut into 3cm chunks

sea salt

handful of chopped coriander leaves, to garnish

1   Preheat the oven to 200°C/180°C fan/gas 6.

2   Heat half the oil in an ovenproof casserole dish and then soften the onion for 5 minutes over a medium heat.

3   Add in the rice, courgette, pepper and curry paste, then stir in the lime zest, coconut milk and 250ml boiling water.

4   Bring to the boil, then put the lid on the dish and bake for 20 minutes.

5   In the meantime, brown the chicken in a frying pan in the remaining coconut oil for about 3 minutes over a medium-high heat. Add to the pot, stir well to combine, then return to the oven to cook for a further 20 minutes, until the rice is nice and fluffy. Add the lime juice, season to taste, and sprinkle over some coriander to serve.

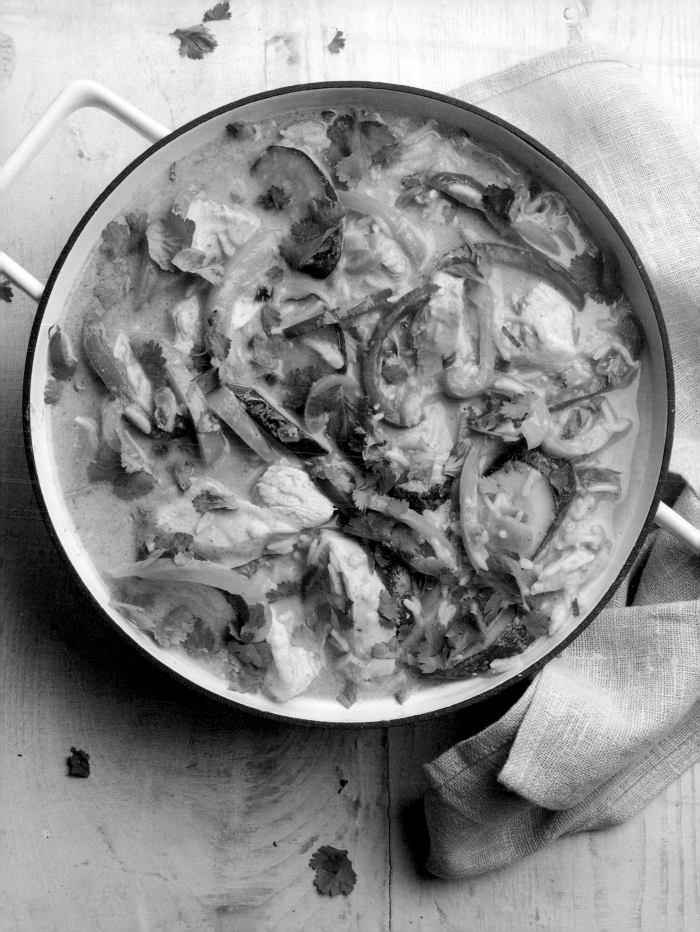

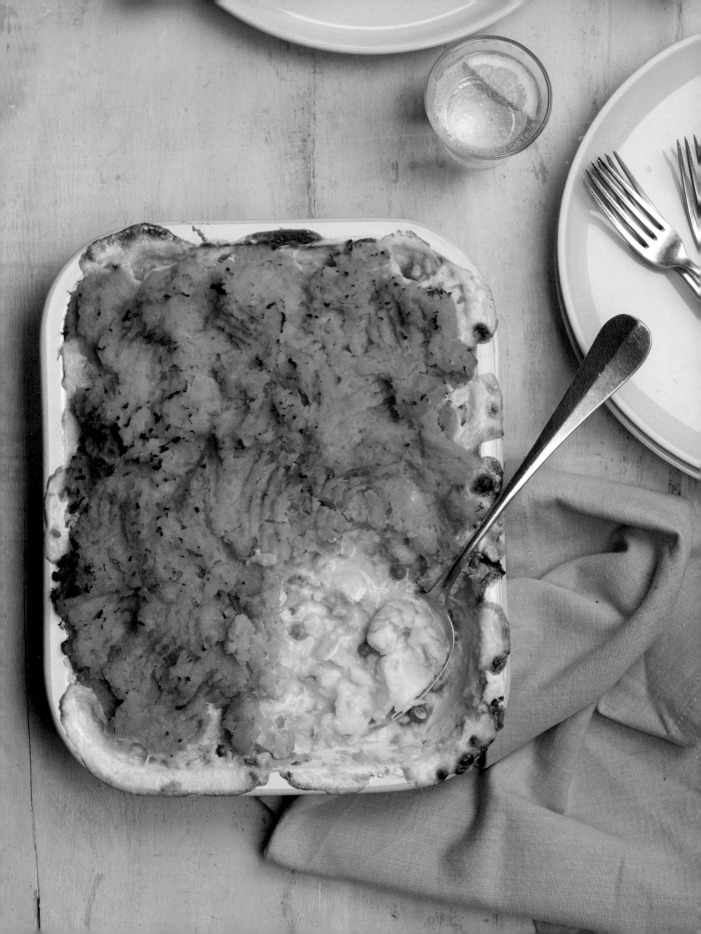

MY FAMILY'S FAVOURITE FISH PIE

My grandad insisted that I set up my own restaurant selling this fish pie – he reckons it's the best he's ever had. I buy frozen fish for this dish as it is a lot more cost-effective.

900g swede, peeled and cut into
   2cm chunks

2 large sweet potatoes, peeled and
   cut into 2cm chunks (around 600g)

1 tbsp butter

2 tbsp olive oil

1 onion, peeled and roughly chopped

1 small garlic clove, peeled and
   crushed

2 tsp English mustard

2 tbsp plain flour

400ml full-fat milk or nut milk (the
   smoked fish will override any
   flavour from the milk)

4 smoked haddock fillets, skinless, cut
   into 5cm chunks

2 salmon fillets, skinless, cut into 5cm
   chunks

3 white fish fillets, skinless

100g raw peeled king prawns

OR

2 frozen bags of good-quality fish pie
   mix (800g in total), defrosted and
   patted dry

350g frozen peas

sea salt and freshly ground black
   pepper

1   Preheat the oven to 200°C/180°C fan/gas 6.

2   Cook all the root vegetables in a large saucepan of boiling water for about 20 minutes, until soft. Drain thoroughly. Now add the butter and mash until lovely and smooth.

3   In the meantime, add the olive oil, onion and garlic to a large saucepan with a pinch of salt and pepper. Fry for 10 minutes over a medium heat, but don't let it burn. Add the mustard and flour and cook for 2 minutes. Gradually pour in the milk, stirring. Bring to the boil, then simmer for about 5 minutes to thicken. Remove from the heat and add all the fish (except the prawns).

4   Spoon the mixture into a 25–30cm ovenproof dish, ensuring the fish is evenly distributed. Scatter the prawns and 4 tablespoons of peas over the top. Season with salt and pepper.

5   Evenly spread the fluffy root vegetable mash over the fish. Place the pie in the oven to cook for a further 15 minutes. In this time you can cook the rest of your peas and any additional greens to accompany your fish pie.

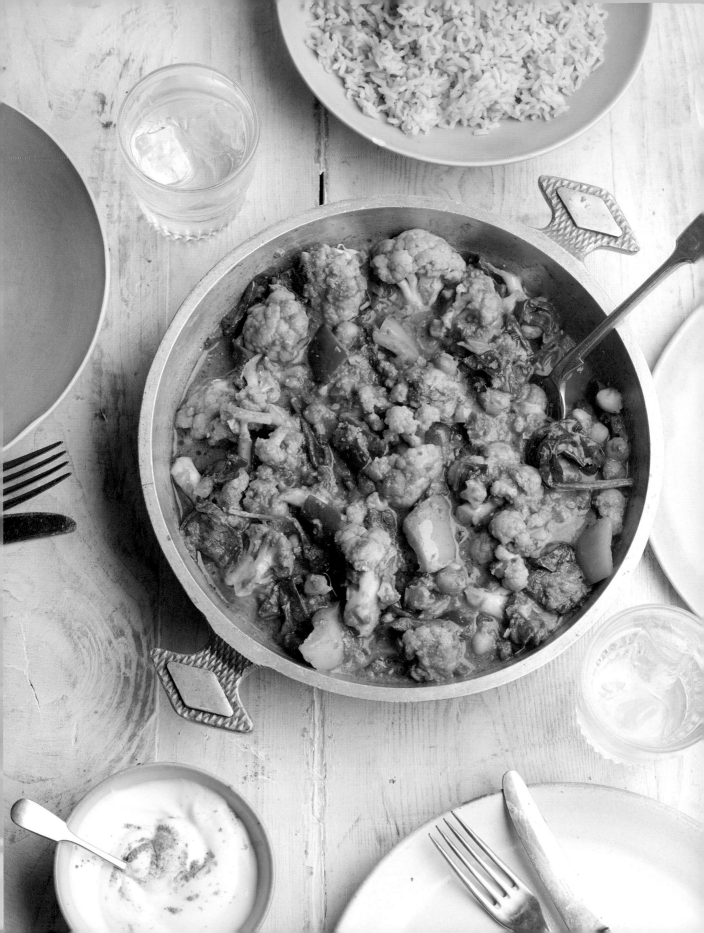

ONE-POT CAULIFLOWER CURRY

You don't always need meat to create a delicious dish, but you certainly need flavour. This is great for entertaining, especially if you're cooking for vegetarian friends.

1 tbsp coconut oil

2 onions, peeled and roughly chopped

1 cauliflower, broken into little florets

2 red, yellow or orange peppers, deseeded and cut into 2cm chunks

2 garlic cloves, peeled and crushed

1 tsp ginger purée

2 heaped tbsp curry powder (mild, medium or hot)

1 tsp ground cumin

1 x 400g tin of chickpeas, drained and rinsed

2 x 400g tins of tomatoes

250g wholegrain or basmati rice, rinsed

250g natural yoghurt

125g bag of baby spinach

sea salt and freshly ground black pepper

1   Add the coconut oil to a large saucepan and add the onion, cauliflower, peppers, garlic, ginger, curry powder and cumin. Let them cook over a medium heat, covered, for about 10 minutes, stirring every now and then until slightly brown and starting to soften.

2   Add the chickpeas and tinned tomatoes and stir again. Cover, reduce the heat to medium-low and let this gently simmer for 20 minutes.

3   Place the rice in a saucepan and cover with cold water. Bring up to the boil, then cover the pan and simmer over a gentle heat for 15–25 minutes (the wholegrain rice needs longer).

4   Now stir the yoghurt into the curry. Let the curry continue to simmer for an additional 20 minutes, adding the spinach and seasoning, to taste, in the final 10 minutes.

5   Drain the rice and plate up in bowls topped with your cauliflower curry.

NOT-SO-NAUGHTY NACHOS WITH HOMEMADE TEX-MEX DIPS

4-6

Enjoy this Mexican platter without the guilt. Using wholemeal pittas instead of tortilla chips and making your own guacamole and salsa is so much healthier.

6 wholemeal pittas, halved horizontally and opened, then cut into triangular quarters
100g jar of sliced jalapeños
150g mozzarella, grated
1 x 210g tin of kidney beans, drained and rinsed
sea salt and freshly ground black pepper

FOR THE GUACAMOLE
2 avocados
2 spring onions, diced
juice of ½ lime
2 tbsp chopped coriander
several drops of Tabasco

FOR THE SALSA
2 tomatoes, deseeded and roughly chopped
¼ red onion, very finely diced
1 tsp olive oil
½ garlic clove, very finely chopped
½ tbsp lime juice

FOR THE SOURED CREAM
100g Greek yoghurt or soured cream
small handful of chives, finely chopped
½ tsp garlic salt

1   First prepare all your Tex-Mex dips. For the guacamole, peel and stone the avocados, roughly chop, and mix with all the other ingredients, squashing gently with a fork and stirring so all the ingredients are evenly distributed. For the salsa, add all the ingredients together and stir, then do the same for the soured cream. Season to taste.

3   Preheat your grill. Place the pitta triangles flat on a tray lined with baking paper or foil and place under the grill until nearly crisp – the time this takes will vary depending on your grill, so keep a close eye on them. Top with the jalapeños, mozzarella and kidney beans and put under the grill for a further few minutes until the cheese has melted.

4   Remove the nachos and gently tower them on top of each other, ensuring you don't leave behind any of the beans. Then either power the dips on top or have them on the side and get stuck in.

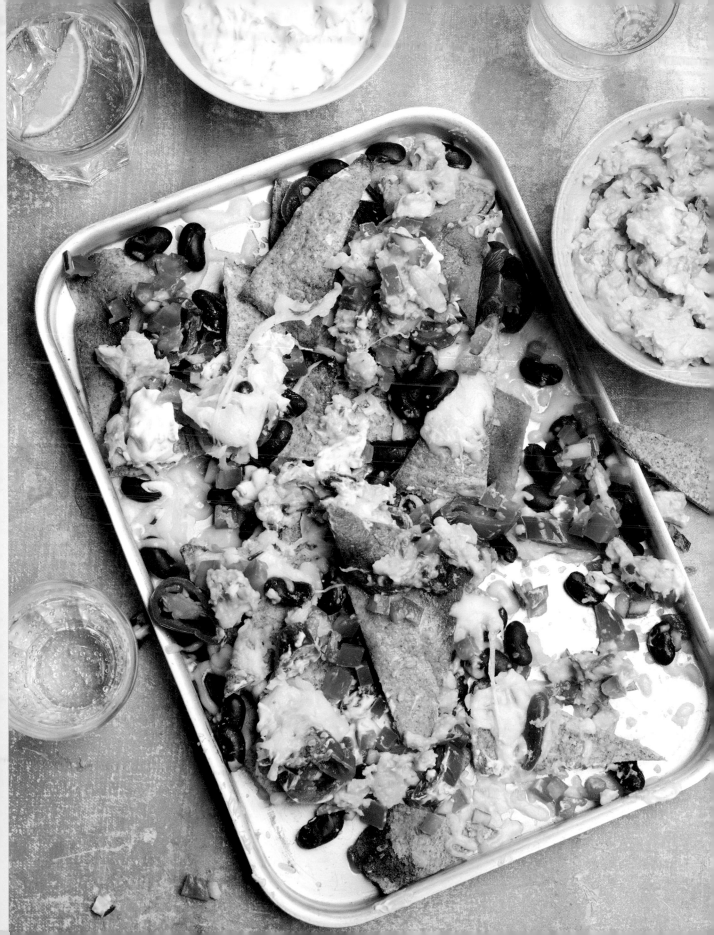

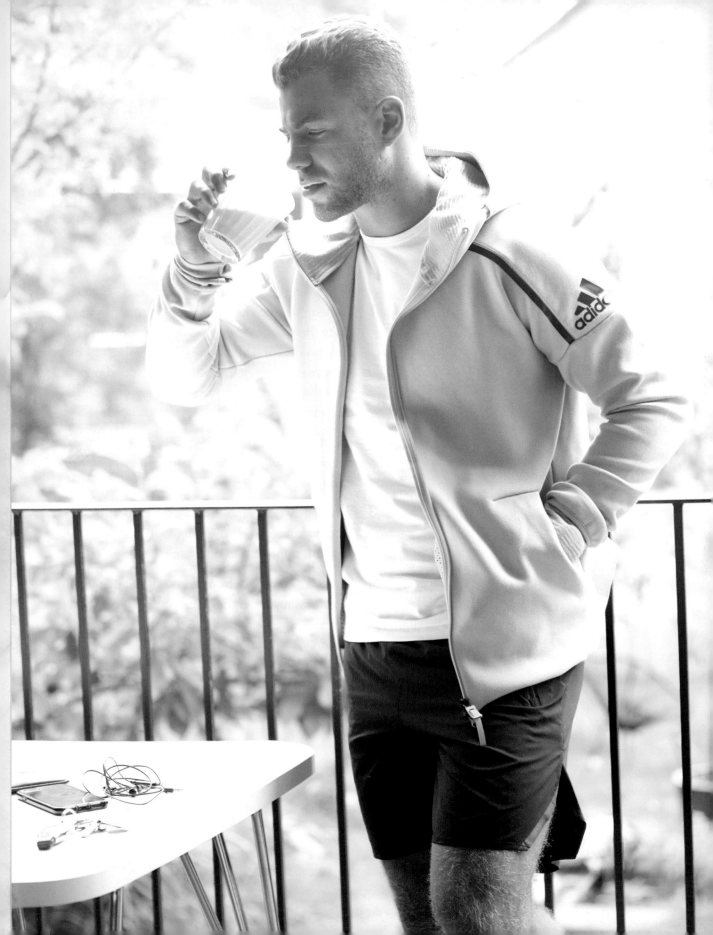

DRINKS & SWEET TREATS

We all need a sweet fix sometimes!

No matter how healthy you are, or healthy you become, there will be days where nothing satisfies you unless it is sweet. If you're one of those people who feels hungry all the time, my smoothies and juices are perfect for packing in some of your ten a day. Alcohol seems to be the hardest thing for people to cut down on when they're trying to lead a healthier lifestyle, so I've created some refined sugar-free cocktails for you to enjoy to make getting your body and mind into tip-top shape less of a sacrifice.

RED VELVET BEETROOT CAKES

9 CAKES

Everyone needs an indulgent treat now and again – it's even better when I know I'm enjoying something that's both indulgent and free from refined sugar. That's exactly what these cakes are, indulgent without the guilt!

2 large raw beetroots, washed, peeled and grated (about 300g)

2 medium eggs

1 tsp vanilla extract

1 tsp ground cinnamon, plus extra for dusting

140g ground almonds

4 tbsp raw cacao powder

1 tsp baking powder

3 tbsp coconut oil, melted

2 tbsp maple syrup or honey, to sweeten

pinch of sea salt

4 tbsp Greek yoghurt

extra-thick Greek yoghurt, to serve

1   Preheat the oven to 200°C/180°C fan/gas 6. Line a muffin tin with 9 paper cases.

2   Blend all the ingredients together in a large bowl until a smooth batter forms and distribute evenly into the muffin cases.

3   Cook for about 20 minutes.

4   Once cooked, let the muffins cool completely before eating. To serve, top each cake with a teaspoon of extra-thick Greek yoghurt and dust with cinnamon.

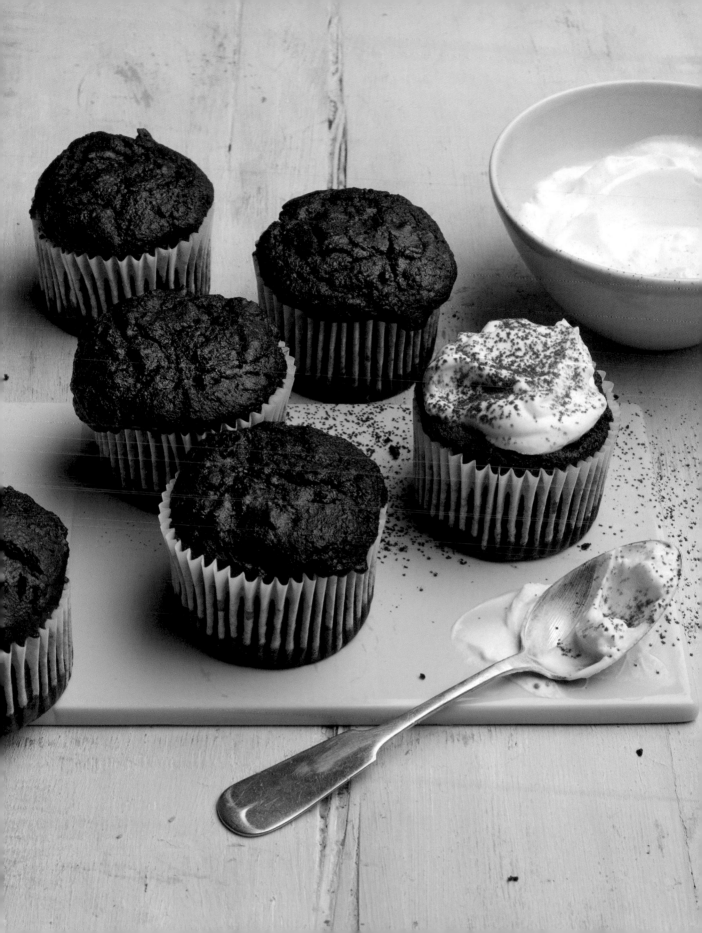

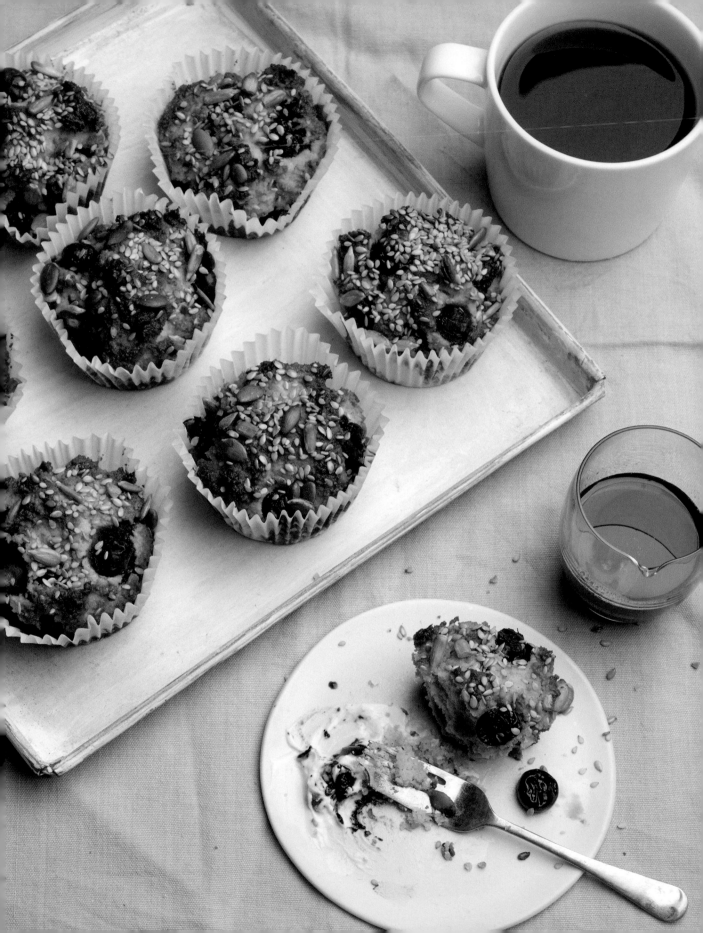

BURSTING BREAKFAST MUFFINS

12 MUFFINS

The sweetness from these muffins comes from the spices and the bursting blueberries. I love eating these with a cup of tea.

300g ground almonds
2 large eggs
1 tbsp Greek yoghurt
1 scant tsp baking powder
2 tbsp maple syrup or honey, plus
    extra to serve
3 tbsp coconut oil, melted
200g blueberries
1 tsp vanilla extract
1 tsp ground cinnamon
1 tsp grated nutmeg
2 tbsp mixed seeds or pumpkin
    seeds
extra-thick Greek yoghurt, to serve

1   Preheat the oven to 200°C/180°C fan/gas 6. Line a muffin tin with 12 paper cases.

2   Add all the ingredients to a large bowl and whisk together until smooth.

3   Distribute evenly into the cases.

4   Cook in the oven for 25 minutes. Now stick the kettle on!

5   Serve with a dollop of Greek yoghurt and a drizzle of maple syrup.

GET-UP-AND-GO BREAKFAST PROTEIN SMOOTHIE

This shake can occasionally be a substitute for breakfast as it includes protein, oats, fruit and good fats – all elements that work together to keep us full and give us energy until midday. Ideally, drink this prior to a morning workout or straight after, not in the evening.

30g scoop of good-quality protein powder (flavour is your choice)
200ml nut milk
30g rolled oats
1 banana
4 whole walnuts
small handful of spinach
4 ice cubes

1   Simply add all the ingredients to a blender and blitz until smooth.

2   Pour into a tall glass and enjoy.

Left to right: Green Super Smoothie, Get-up-and-go Breakfast Protein Smoothie, Full of Berries Smoothie

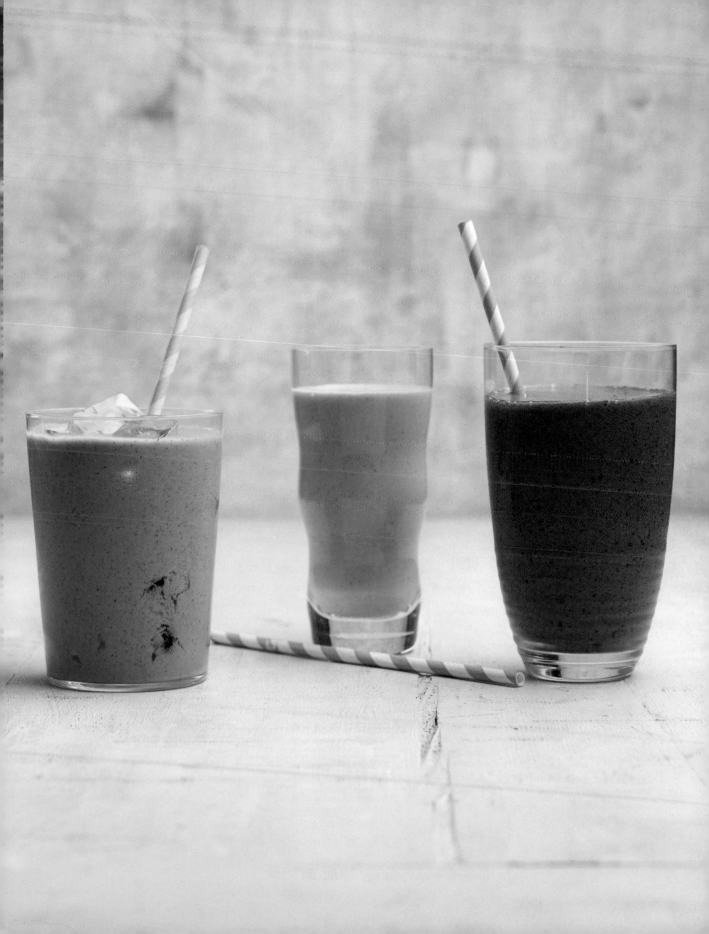

CONNIE'S COCONUT COLADA

Connie helped me out with this one. She wanted to create something creamy with coconuts, so a coconut colada it is – the perfect after-dinner cocktail with friends.

2 shots of rum (I like coconut rum best with this) (60ml)
100ml coconut cream
150ml coconut water
1½ tsp vanilla extract
1 pineapple ring (in its own juices or water, not syrup)
1 tsp honey
pinch of grated nutmeg
6 ice cubes

1 Add all the ingredients to a blender and blitz up until slushy.

2 Poor into two glasses, sit back, relax and enjoy.

Left to right: Grapefruit and Gin Cucumber Cooler, Elderflower and Prosecco Fizz, Skinny Cranberry Cosmo

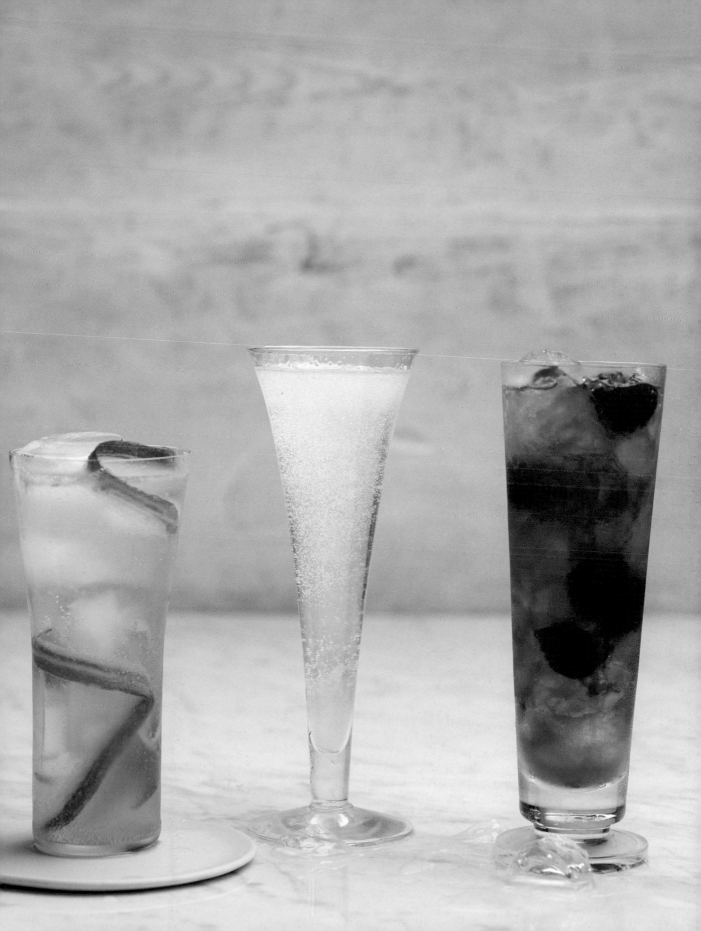

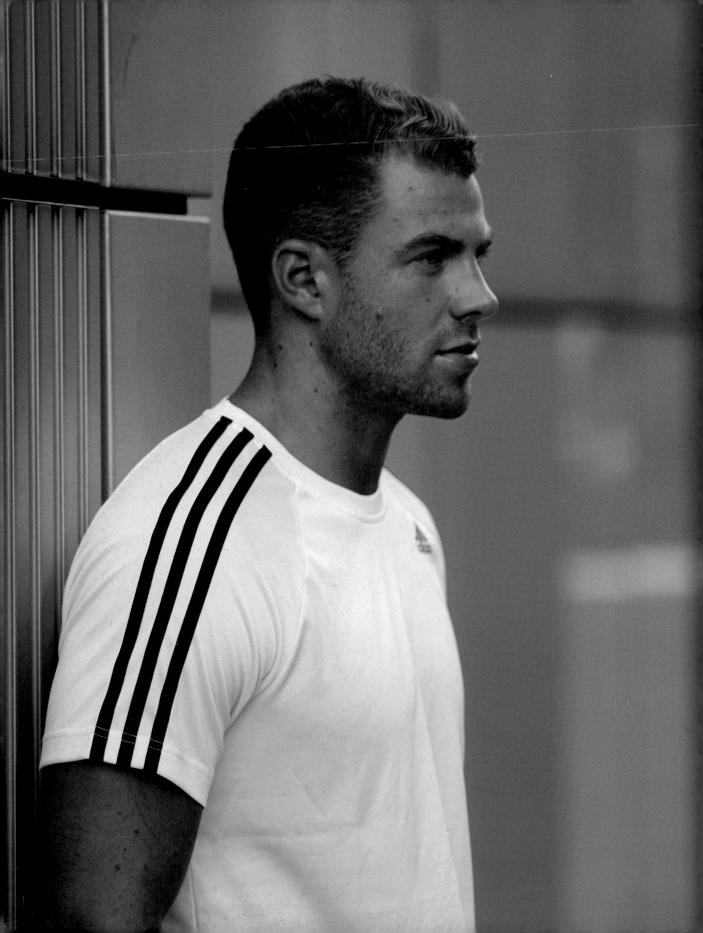

CHAPTER 4

MAINTAINING YOUR GOAL

MEASURE YOUR PROGRESS

Measuring your progress is mega-important for staying motivated and feeling good about your new healthy lifestyle. You want to feel strong, proud and determined every step of the way, and that only comes with solid proof that your hard work is paying off! A glance in the mirror won't cut it, especially if you're looking at your body every day, and guessing isn't satisfying enough.

By now you'll have decided on your first goal. Now you need a way of measuring it that works for you so you can tick off the milestones and move on to a whole new goal.

Just like exercise and nutrition, the measuring method that works for you could be totally different to what works for someone else. How you choose to measure your progress is very personal. For example, I very rarely use scales because my weight fluctuates so often, and I don't consider it to be an accurate indication of how close I am to reaching my goals at any one time. But for some people, this approach is comforting and familiar, and it works for them.

Here I'll be highlighting the pros and cons of different measuring techniques and outlining several options that I recommend when it comes to keeping tabs on your progress. The key factors you should keep track of are:

- Body fat percentage
- Body shape
- Muscle definition
- Internal health

All these markers are far more indicative of improvements in your health (not to mention your appearance) than your actual weight.

WEIGHING SCALES

The traditional way to measure progress (outdated to my mind) is by using weighing scales. Like I say, I'm not a fan. The scales only consider one factor. What they don't show is how much of that weight is water, fat or muscle. You may have made leaps and strides in terms of progress, but that won't be reflected on the scales, which has the effect of demotivating you.

MUSCLE WEIGHS MORE THAN FAT
You've probably heard this said, and what it means is that muscle is more dense than fat – so if you had a cube of muscle and the same size cube of fat side by side, the muscle would weight more than the fat. What this means for your body is that two people can weigh exactly the same, but one will have larger muscles and less fat, be healthier and appear smaller, and one will have smaller muscles and more fat, be less healthy and appear larger.

So remember, you may lose pounds of fat and gain muscle and look completely different, but you could still weigh the same on the scales if the amount of fat you've lost is the same as the amount of muscle you have gained.

Don't let this put you off building muscle, either. We've already touched on how vital lean muscle is for our strength, stability and body function. It's much healthier to focus on building up this necessary muscle than it is to weigh as little as possible on the scales. If in doubt, go back to the toning chapter to reacquaint yourself with the facts. Then ditch those scales!

PROGRESS PHOTOS

Taking photos of yourself might make you feel vain or just plain uncomfortable, but it's one of the most effective methods of measuring progress when it comes to your body.

My sister uses this method and has found it really useful; it's kept her motivated and allows her to see at the tap of a button just how far she's come on her weight-loss journey. Sometimes (most of the time!) numbers on a bit of paper just don't have the same effect as a before and after picture.

If you're feeling brave and you're prepared for any personal comments or repercussions (I'd recommend taking photos from the neck down for this reason so should your image get circulated more widely, you're not identifiable) you might even want to share your progress with family and friends on social media or with an online fitness or weight-loss community that you're part of. Many people find sharing their progress motivates them, because they're publicly committing to a healthy way of life. It's so much harder to back-pedal once you've essentially made a public declaration of intent, especially if you get congratulated on your progress on the way! Transformation pictures are also a massive hit on social media because of their power to inspire others.

If you'd like to try this method of measuring your progress, I'd advise taking pictures of yourself in your underwear no more frequently than every four weeks – enough time for noticeable changes to take place to your body. Always aim to use the same mirror and lighting each time you take a photo, as both of these factors can impact what we see. Those are the pros! The con: this method focuses on appearance and not health. A photo can't show you whether the fat around your organs has reduced (although this is usually a natural by-product of a healthier lifestyle).

MEASURING TAPE

This is another old-fashioned method, but it's a goodie if your goal is to lose a couple of inches around your waist, back, bum, tummy, arms or thighs or to gain weight healthily. What it won't do is tell you how much of the weight lost or gained is fat or muscle – you'll need to use another method to work that out. Taking measurements this way also tends to be more time-consuming than taking photos, but if numbers and collecting data is your thing, give it a go. Just make sure you're consistent with where you place the measuring tape so you can make a proper comparison.

MEASURING BODY FAT PERCENTAGE WITH EQUIPMENT

This is – hands down – the most accurate way of figuring out how much progress you're making. Use this equipment in conjunction with guideline healthy body fat percentages for men and women (see below), which will help you figure out realistic body fat aims, depending on your personal goals.

MEN	WOMEN
Essential Fat 2–4%	Essential Fat 9–12%
Athletes 6–13%	Athletes 14–20%
Fitness 14–17%	Fitness 21–24%
Acceptable 18–25%	Acceptable 25–31%
Overweight 26% +	Overweight 32% +

I aim to keep my body fat percentage between 10 and 14 percent – it's the right amount for me and my job and lifestyle. But one person's ambition won't be shared by everyone and what's realistic and feasible for one person isn't possible for another – we all have different goals, priorities and body shapes. Regardless of that, you should know that having SOME fat on our body is vital for organ function and the production of hormones. I would never recommend anyone be in the Essential Fat category for long periods of time, just as I'd never recommend anyone be in the Overweight category. Again, it's all about balance.

If you're unsure of your body fat percentage, you should definitely consider checking it out every so often using either body fat calipers, which pinch the fat and give you a measurement that you compare with figures on a chart, or a body fat scale or monitor that sends a current through your body. Both of these methods are fairly accurate and will give you an idea of where you're at, and they're affordable too – great if you're on a tight budget or just want to do your measuring at home.

But the very best way to measure your body fat percentage is by visiting a Bod Pod. This device calculates not only your body fat percentage, but the percentage of fat around the organs. It's pretty remarkable and super accurate. The only downfall is the price tag: it can be around £75 for a scan, but if you're serious about your body and health and have the money, it's worth every penny to get you started on your goals.

NUTRITIONISTS AND OTHER OPTIONS

Regardless of how healthy and fit we become, we can still have niggles or issues with our body, such as bloating, poor digestion, bad skin, bad breath and headaches, which can be so frustrating when you've worked so hard. If you're in this position, I really sympathise, and I'd strongly advise that you visit a nutritionist or a doctor with dietary experience for further tests and support. Everyone deserves good health, especially when they've worked hard for it.

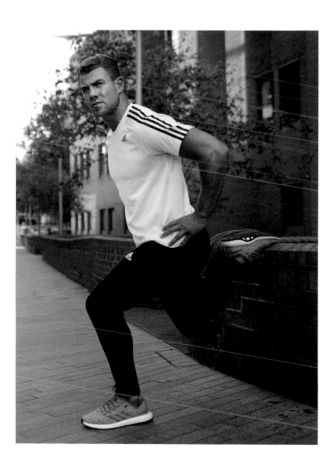

MAINTAIN YOUR GOAL

It is an amazing achievement to drop a dress size in time for a wedding or get a toned tummy ready for your trip to Ibiza, but a lot of us fall down when it comes to maintaining these goals. I rarely hear the words, 'I'm going to get in shape this summer, and stay that way all year round,' or, 'I'm going to get to my healthy weight for this wedding and make sure I never put the extra weight back on,' but that's what we ought to be aiming for: fewer quick fixes and more long-term lifestyle changes. That way healthy living becomes a natural part of day-to-day life and you don't have the pressure or stress of suddenly needing to join the gym and go hardcore on your diet on 1 January after too many mince pies.

Wouldn't it be nice to not have to worry about any of this at all? One day, you may not have to. Consistency and better choices will lead to your new healthier lifestyle, and because you'll be feeling so good, there'll be no going back.

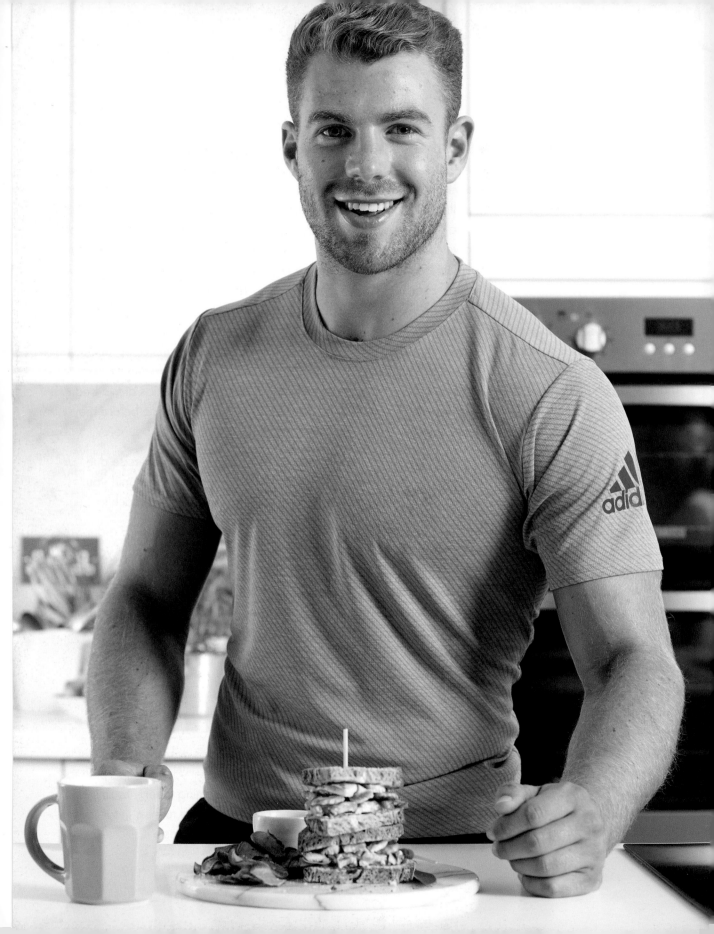

YOU'RE READY

Now, before you put the book down and get stuck in to your no excuses, no regrets, body-and-mind revolution, let's recap:

Introduction: Remember my journey? I realised my goal and decided who I wanted to be and how I wanted to look, feel and think, and I gave you a few ideas as to how you could start your own journey to healthy living.

Chapter 1 – Realising Your Goal: Kick start your journey with a realistic, measurable goal that you really care about and draw up your plan for realising it.

Chapter 2 – Now Get Moving: Step-by-step exercises for your personal work-out plan.

Chapter 3 – Fuel Your Fitness: Tuck into my nutritious and delicious recipes.

Chapter 4 – Maintaining Your Goal: Track the changes you're making every step of the way, pledge to maintain your original goal and decide on the next one to keep you motivated and sustain your new, healthy way of life.

Don't forget, I'm just like you; I've experienced frustration, temptation and self-doubt, but I picked myself up, focused on my health, pushed myself and put myself out there to get fitter and healthier than I've ever been before. The focus, happiness and success that followed was a natural side effect. I've written this book because I want you to feel the same way.

So keep this guide close and let it motivate you every step of the way.

Good luck with your journey!

Bradley

RECIPES INDEX

ACKNOWLEDGEMENTS

There are so many people to thank; from my days as a young footballer right up to this book being published, I've had endless support and encouragement from so many people. To name just a few...

Firstly, I would like to say a huge thank you to the team at at HarperCollins for seeing the potential in this book. You've become a huge part in helping me to reach my goal to inspire and educate people around the world.

I'd also like to thank my manager Issy Lloyd for her ongoing support and hard work, her dedication to her job continues to inspire me.

I'm extremely grateful for my family. I'm so lucky to have such a positive support network around me. From my grandparents to my little cousins, they're my number one fans and are always cheering me on.

I'd like to thank my sister Connie. Your weight loss transformation in particular has allowed us to inspire and motivate thousands of people to do the same. Your commitment to your new lifestyle has proven that it is possible to realistically sustain a healthier way of life, I wouldn't have been able to showcase this without documenting your own personal journey.

Last but not least, thank you to my clients and followers. Right from the early days you've helped me to grow as a professional. I start each day with you in mind, you keep me focused and determined to continue to learn in my profession. My role to motivate and encourage you has come full circle.